# Diabetic Cooking Made Easy

A Beginner's Guide
to Healthy
Meals at Home

American Diabetes
Association

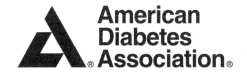

**American
Diabetes
Association**®

*Director, Book Operations*, Victor Van Beuren; *Managing Editor, Books*, John Clark; *Associate Director, Book Marketing*, Annette Reape; *Acquisitions Editor*, Jaclyn Konich; *Copyeditor*, Wendy Martin-Shuma; *Composition*, Jeska Horgan-Kobelski; *Cover Design*, Vis-à-vis Creative; *Stock Photography*, Adobe Stock; *Printer*, Versa Press.

Printed in the United States of America

1 3 5 7 9 10 8 6 4 2

The suggestions and information contained in this publication are generally consistent with the Standards of Medical Care in Diabetes and other policies of the American Diabetes Association, but they do not represent the policy or position of the Association or any of its boards or committees. Reasonable steps have been taken to ensure the accuracy of the information presented. However, the American Diabetes Association cannot ensure the safety or efficacy of any product or service described in this publication. Individuals are advised to consult a physician or other appropriate health care professional before undertaking any diet or exercise program or taking any medication referred to in this publication. Professionals must use and apply their own professional judgment, experience, and training and should not rely solely on the information contained in this publication before prescribing any diet, exercise, or medication. The American Diabetes Association—its officers, directors, employees, volunteers, and members—assumes no responsibility or liability for personal or other injury, loss, or damage that may result from the suggestions or information in this publication.

Jo Mandelson, MS, RDN, conducted the internal review of this book to ensure that it meets American Diabetes Association guidelines.

∞ The paper in this publication meets the requirements of the ANSI Standard Z39.48-1992 (permanence of paper).

ADA titles may be purchased for business or promotional use or for special sales. To purchase more than 50 copies of this book at a discount, or for custom editions of this book with your logo, contact the American Diabetes Association at the address below or at booksales@diabetes.org.

American Diabetes Association
2451 Crystal Drive, Suite 900
Arlington, VA 22202

DOI: 10.2337/9781580407656

Library of Congress Control Number: 2020942630

# CONTENTS

# Introduction

Whether you are just learning to manage a new diabetes diagnosis or have been living with diabetes for years, this book will help guide you in making easy, healthy choices that fit your lifestyle. The simple instructions in this book break down the basics of cooking for 1 or even 10 people while maximizing your food budget.

In this Introduction, you will find resources for discovering great recipes and how-to videos to help with finding groceries, if that is a struggle for you and your family. Chapter 1 includes a guide to the must-have kitchen tools that are essential for easy, home cooking, and you'll learn how to set yourself up for success with the right recipes: including learning how to follow the recipes and, most important, how to prepare food safely. There is also a glossary of cooking terms included in Chapter 1.

Throughout the rest of the book, we get busy shopping, cooking, and learning how to make the basics, from chicken to vegetables and everything in between. We will teach you to shop, prep, cook, store, thaw, and reheat, while learning to save time and money along the way. There are also lists of measurements and conversions at the end of the book, with a helpful substitutions guide.

*Diabetic Cooking Made Easy* is for anyone who wants healthy cooking to be easy and tasty, and who doesn't want an ingredient list that is 20 items long, filled with things you've never heard of. The recipes and information are presented in a simple and easy-to-understand format and will help you thrive in the kitchen and in life.

# RESOURCES

The recipes in this book are simple and include detailed instructions to help you though the process. We have also provided a glossary of terms and simple tips to help you out, but if there are terms, cooking methods, equipment, or techniques that you are not familiar with, the following online resources can be helpful:

*Diabetes Food Hub:* From the nutrition experts at the American Diabetes Association, Diabetes Food Hub is the premier food and cooking destination for people living with diabetes and their families. **https://www.diabetesfoodhub.org**

*U.S. Department of Agriculture (USDA):* MyPlate Kitchen from the USDA provides recipes and resources to support building healthy and budget-friendly meals. USDA also offers a mobile app to help search recipes, food groups, nutrition information, and other great resources on the go. **https://www.choosemyplate.gov**

*YouTube:* YouTube is a free resource filled with millions of videos on any subject, including many instructional videos on cooking

## CHEF TIP

When using the Internet to look for cooking help or recipes, be sure to use sites that are reputable and have expertise in that area. Not all recipes online are tested by the recipe creators, and the dish may not turn out properly. If you are new to cooking, you may think a cooking failure is your fault when it is actually the recipe's fault. Don't get discouraged! Start with the recipes in this book and from the American Diabetes Association online (**https://www.diabetesfoodhub.org**), and practice! Once you learn some basic skills, go exploring for new recipes online. You can always pick up new cookbooks in bookstores or at the library so you can try out recipes that you know have been tested. And remember: Have fun!

and food prep. You can search using phrases about specific skills, such as "how to mince an onion," or follow trusted channels such as America's Test Kitchen, Epicurious, Food52, or Tastemade, to name a few. **https://www.youtube.com**

*Feeding America:* Feeding America is the largest hunger relief organization in the U.S. and has an online resource guide that offers delicious, healthy recipes for lower-income families created by food banks from all across the country. You can also sort the recipes by food group and find kid-friendly recipes. **https://hungerandhealth.feedingamerica.org/healthy-recipes**

# CHAPTER 1

## Getting Started

Cooking is a skill, not an art. Often we think we have to be naturally talented at cooking or have TV-personality passion to get in the kitchen and create. That isn't true. With simple instructions, easy-to-follow recipes, and some basic equipment, you can make meals and snacks for the whole week that are budget friendly, quick, and delicious.

## ESSENTIAL KITCHEN TOOLS

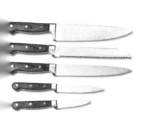

It all starts with the right tools. And the good news is, you don't need every kitchen gadget you see on late-night infomercials; you just need some basic tools that will make prepping and cooking a breeze. You don't have to go out and get all of these items at once, either. Start with one or two, and then build your kitchen toolbox over time.

Here are some essential tools to have in your kitchen:

*Knives.* Most important, you will need a good, sharp chef's knife. If you want to add a couple of other knives that are helpful in the kitchen, a serrated knife and a paring knife are the next two most important after the chef's knife.

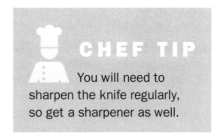

**CHEF TIP**

You will need to sharpen the knife regularly, so get a sharpener as well.

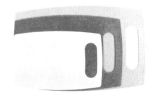

*Cutting board.* A grippy, plastic one is best for easiest cleaning and cutting safety. We recommend having more than one cutting board. For food safety, it's best to designate one cutting board for cutting raw meat only.

## CHEF TIP

If the cutting board doesn't have grips on it to keep it in place, wet a paper towel and put it under the cutting board so it doesn't slide around.

*Measuring cups and spoons.* Measuring tools are especially critical for baking, but also for ensuring portion control.

*Pots and pans.* For cooking on the stove, you will need a nonstick skillet (also called a frying pan), a saucepan, and a stock pot (also called a soup pot)

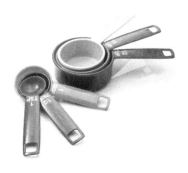

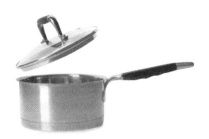

*Baking dishes.* For cooking in the oven, you'll need one or more sheet pans (also called a baking sheet or cookie sheet pan), a casserole dish (9 × 13 or 8 × 8 inches; glass is best), and a nonstick muffin pan.

*Refrigerator and freezer-safe storage containers.* Glass containers are best and are reusable, but plastic containers and disposable freezer bags work well, too. Mason jars make great storage containers that are also easy to take on the go. You can typically purchase these as a set, with the jar, lid, and sealing ring included.

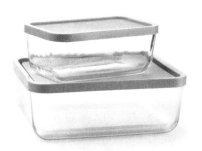

*Other utensils and tools:* Bowls (in a variety of sizes from small to large); heat-proof rubber spatula; whisk; tongs; peeler; spatula for turning items (we recommend a fish turner); can opener; mesh colander (for draining or rinsing items); box grater; and digital meat thermometer.

*Helpful but not essential tools:* Blender; food processor; slow cooker; immersion blender; microplane/zester; and potato masher.

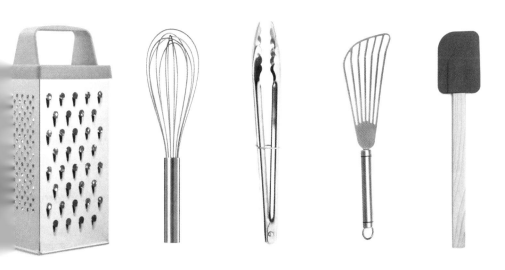

# HOW TO USE A RECIPE

When starting with a new recipe, you must read the whole thing before you are ready to cook. In fact, you should read it thoroughly even before making your grocery list. The recipe will not only tell you the list of ingredients and the amounts you need to make the recipe, but it will also provide the directions you must follow to cook properly, any equipment you'll need, the pre-steps (such as thawing an item or preheating an oven), as well as the prep time, cook time, how much the recipe will make (usually called the "yield"), and serving size and nutritional information. It is vital to read the whole recipe—ingredients and directions—before making your grocery list, so that you not only know how much of each ingredient to buy, but also to ensure you have all of the right equipment to make the recipe. You are not going to be able to make a slow-cooker recipe if you don't have a slow cooker, right?

Once you understand the ingredients and directions and have shopped for the groceries, it's time to get set up for cooking. Follow these steps for success:

1. Gather all of the ingredients and equipment you will need for the recipe so that you have everything in reach before beginning.
2. Take any pre-steps required, such as washing produce or preheating an oven.
3. Read the directions for any hidden ingredients such as water or seasoning that may have been left out of the ingredients (Note: great recipes won't make that mistake, but some do) or terms or methods you may not understand. Look up these unfamiliar terms or methods if they are not defined.
4. Measure each ingredient as called for in the recipe and place in a prep bowl or organize on a baking sheet. Double-check your recipe

to make sure you have everything and have taken all of the pre-steps before you start to cook.

5. Follow the instructions for cooking the recipe.

To ensure you are meeting the nutritional requirements in your meal plan, measure the portion size according to what the recipe lists as the serving size. For example, a recipe may yield 4 cups total, with the serving size as 1 cup. The nutrition information is listed by serving size, so the calories, fat, cholesterol, sodium, potassium, carbohydrate, protein, and phosphorus listed will be based on that 1-cup serving size. If you eat the entire recipe, you have consumed four times the serving-size amount, so you should multiply all of the nutrition information by four.

## FOOD SAFETY BASICS

Keeping yourself safe during cooking is essential. Certain food and cooking practices may pose health risks that can be as mild as an upset stomach or as severe as death. Cooking surfaces and equipment that are easy to clean and sanitize are essential, and following cooking guidelines for internal temperatures of meat, poultry, seafood, and eggs is vital. It is also important to keep yourself (mainly your hands) and your cooking surfaces clean and to avoid cross-contaminating ingredients (e.g., don't cut ready-to-eat vegetables on the same cutting board where you just cut raw chicken).

Follow these basic guidelines to stay safe and healthy in the kitchen:

1. Store:

- Store your ingredients at the proper temperatures (store cold foods in the refrigerator and frozen foods in the freezer). Check ingredients for use-by dates and signs of freshness before cooking.

- Separate raw meat, poultry, seafood, and eggs from other ingredients and keep them below other food items in your refrigerator or freezer, so they can't drip on ready-to-eat foods (foods that do not require further cooking).

- Do not thaw ingredients on the countertop; they will be at a temperature that is too warm for too long, which may promote bacterial growth. Thaw in the refrigerator, under cold running water, or in the microwave (foods thawed in cold running water and the microwave should be cooked immediately).

- Marinate foods in the refrigerator.

2. Clean:

- Wash your hands regularly with hot, soapy water before and after cooking, between tasks (especially between handling raw meat, poultry, seafood, or eggs), or if you sneeze, cough, or touch anything other than your food or food-contact surface.

- Wash all food-contact surfaces with hot, soapy water between tasks, like when you move from cutting raw meat, poultry, seafood, or eggs to cutting ready-to-eat foods such as vegetables. It is also a good practice to have a separate cutting board for raw meat, poultry, seafood, or eggs and a separate cutting board for all other foods.

- Keep your shopping bags off of the counter where you will be cooking, and be sure to clean your cooking space before you start cooking.

- Wash **all** produce. (See "Produce Prep and Storage" on page 40 for tips on washing produce.)
- Wash your sink regularly.

3. Cook properly:

- All foods should be cooked to the proper internal temperature to ensure food safety. 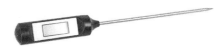 Use a quick-read or digital thermometer to ensure proper temperatures of food, taking the temperature in the thickest part of the ingredient. The U.S. Department of Agriculture (USDA) recommends the following temperatures for safety:

  - Beef roasts and steaks: 145°F
  - Pork: 145°F
  - All poultry (chicken, turkey, game hens): 165°F
  - Ground meat (not including turkey, see poultry): 160°F
  - Eggs: Cook until the yolks and whites are firm. Casseroles and other dishes containing eggs should be cooked to 160°F.
  - Fish: 145°F
  - Sauces, soups, and gravy: Bring to a boil when reheating.
  - Other leftovers: Reheat to 165°F.

# GLOSSARY OF TERMS AND TECHNIQUES

*Bake:* To cook by dry heat, usually in the oven.

*Blanch:* To immerse in rapidly boiling water and allow to cook slightly.

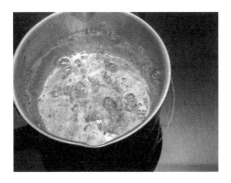

*Boil:* To heat a liquid until bubbles rapidly break continually on the surface (212°F).

*Broil:* To cook under high, direct heat. Ovens typically have a "broil" setting where high heat comes from the top of the oven only.

*Chop:* To cut into non-uniform pieces with a knife.

*Clove of garlic:* A clove of garlic is one of the many small pieces that make up a whole head of garlic, which is comprised of many cloves attached at the base. The head and cloves have a papery cover. To peel a clove of garlic, press the clove under the flat blade of your knife or under a spatula to crush it slightly and break papery skin, then remove the skin.

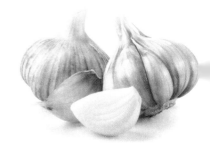

*"Cook to fork tender":* A food is "fork tender" when you pierce it with a fork and the tines enter easily with no resistance. It's important to use a fork and not a knife, since a knife is sharp and may go through the item easier, even if it's not fully cooked.

**Dice:** Dicing is a cutting term that refers to cutting into small blocks. Remember, you don't need perfect cuts, just do your best!

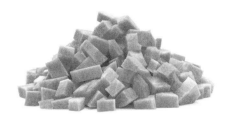

**Small dice:** A small dice is usually around 1/4-inch square.

**Medium dice:** A medium dice is usually around 1/2-inch square.

**Large dice:** A large dice is usually around 3/4-inch square.

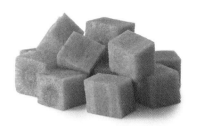

**"Fluff with a fork":** To fluff with a fork means to use a fork to gently stir the food (usually grains such as rice, quinoa, or barley) after it has cooked and rested to release steam and avoid overcooking.

**Pinch:** A pinch of something is the equivalent of about 1/16 of a teaspoon.

**Mince:** Mince is a knife cut that is as small as possible without being puréed.

**Rib of celery:** A rib of celery is one piece of celery from a stalk or head of celery that contains many ribs connected at the bottom by a "heart." Remove the leaves, wash well, and use.

**Roast:** To cook by dry heat in an oven. Roasting is typically done at a higher heat than baking, and the goal is to brown and crisp the exterior of the food.

*Sauté:* To cook the food in a small amount of fat over high heat. Stir frequently to make sure that the food doesn't burn or stick to the pan while sautéing.

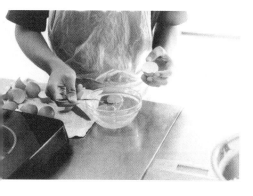

*Separating an egg white from yolk:* Egg whites are the clear part of the egg (albumen) separated from the yellow yolk. There are several methods for separating an egg yolk from the white. Try this method: crack the egg into a small bowl, then carefully scoop out the yolk with a small spoon or a slotted spoon. The white should separate and drip over the side of the spoon (or through the slots) while the yolk remains in the spoon. If you are just using the whites, discard the yolk. You can also buy pasteurized egg whites in a carton in the egg section of the grocery store. The container will have the equivalent measurement of the carton egg whites to a large egg.

*Simmer:* To cook slowly in liquid over low heat at a temperature of about 180°F. The surface of the liquid should barely be bubbling.

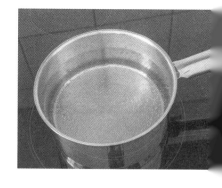

*Thaw and squeeze spinach:* To thaw and squeeze frozen spinach, put the frozen spinach in a mesh colander and run it under very warm water until it is thawed. Then transfer it to a clean kitchen towel or a couple of sheets of stacked strong paper towels and squeeze as much of the liquid out of it as you can. Do this over the colander in case the paper towel rips.

# CHAPTER 2

# Shopping

## TIPS FOR SHOPPING ON A BUDGET

To save time and money in the long run, it is best to spend a little time planning what you will eat in the upcoming week, making a grocery list, and doing some food prep. These steps will ensure that groceries will not go to waste and you won't need to resort to fast food or carry out. To make your life a little easier and your diet healthier, try these "cooking on a budget" tips:

1. Plan what you will eat each week and be realistic about it. You will need cut-up fruits and vegetables, some protein, a starch or two, and some snacks. You will likely eat out one or two meals, so be sure to plan that in your budget.

2. Make a grocery list. This step will keep you on track at the grocery store, and you won't end up with a refrigerator full of groceries and no idea what to do with them.

3. Buy in bulk. You can bring home the bulk items and portion and freeze them (like meat) or store them in your pantry. See more tips for storing food on page 42.

4. Use coupons or a coupon app. Scan the weekly sales at your favorite store and plan your meals around what foods are on sale.

5. Buy frozen vegetables for cooking so they are less likely to go bad in your refrigerator. Choose frozen vegetables with no added sauces or salt (check the ingredients list). (See "Fresh, Frozen, or Canned?" below for more tips on buying vegetables.)

6. Short on time? Many stores offer a "click and collect" option where you can purchase groceries online and schedule them for pickup, usually with no extra fee. Some stores also take SNAP (Supplemental Nutrition Assistance Program) for online ordering and pickup. And by purchasing online, you are less tempted by those tantalizing cookie displays!

7. Buy produce that is in season. It is usually much more afford-able, and because it's in season, it tastes better. For a list of produce seasons, visit https://snaped.fns.usda.gov/seasonal-produce-guide.

8. Buy generic brands. Generic/store-brand products are usually much cheaper than their name-brand counterparts, and their quality is just as good.

## FRESH, FROZEN, OR CANNED?

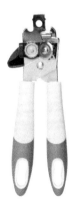

Fresh, frozen, or canned foods can all be perfectly healthy options. Many believe that "fresh is best," but frozen and canned foods are often just as healthy, and they have many advantages. Frozen and canned foods are often cheaper than fresh and have a much longer shelf-life. Knowing when to use which kind and what to look for when purchasing can help save money.

# FRESH

| | Best for... | Not as good for... | What to look for when shopping... |
|---|---|---|---|
| **Vegetables**<br>**Fruit** | Raw dishes like salads; snacking | Fresh vegetables, fruit, and meat can be used in most recipes, but are not always required. Fresh foods have a shorter shelf life, so keep that in mind when shopping and planning meals. | Shop in season, consider ripeness; buy produce that is less ripe if you are using later in the week |
| **Meat/fish** | Quick cooking (no need for thawing) | | Check dates on the package for freshness, longer shelf-life |

# FROZEN

| | Best for... | Not as good for... | What to look for when shopping... |
|---|---|---|---|
| **Vegetables** | Long-cooking dishes like soups or stews, stir-fry, casseroles, steaming, and sautéing | Salads, snacking, roasting | No added sauces or salt; the only ingredient should be the vegetable |
| **Fruit** | Smoothies; cooked fruit like compote; adding to yogurt, oatmeal, etc. | Raw preparation like salads, snacking | No added sugar |
| **Meat/fish** | If thawed first, frozen meat and fish can be used just like fresh | Quick cooking (need time to thaw) | Individually vacuum-sealed cuts, no signs of freezer burn or ice crystals |

| CANNED | Best for... | Not as good for... | What to look for when shopping... |
|---|---|---|---|
| **Vegetables** | Soups and stews, casseroles | Raw dishes, roasting, steaming, or sautéing | No-salt-added, low-sodium, or reduced-sodium; rinse and drain before using to remove more sodium |
| **Fruit** | Snacking; cooked fruit like compote; adding to yogurt, oatmeal, etc. | Raw dishes such as salads | No-sugar-added, canned in water or 100% juice; avoid "canned in heavy syrup" |
| **Meat/fish** | Chicken/tuna salad, burger patties, casseroles, soups | Grilling (unless in burger form), sautéing | Packed in water (not oil), no added flavorings or ingredients, check sodium |

# HOW TO READ A NUTRITION LABEL

## Nutrition Facts

8 servings per container

**Serving size**     **2/3 cup (55g)**

**Amount per serving**

## Calories     230

| | % Daily Value* |
|---|---|
| **Total Fat** 8g | **10%** |
| Saturated Fat 1g | **5%** |
| *Trans* Fat 0g | |
| **Cholesterol** 0mg | **0%** |
| **Sodium** 160mg | **7%** |
| **Total Carbohydrate** 37g | **13%** |
| Dietary Fiber 4g | **14%** |
| Total Sugars 12g | |
| Includes 10g Added Sugars | **20%** |
| **Protein** 3g | |
| Vitamin D 2mcg | 10% |
| Calcium 260mg | 20% |
| Iron 8mg | 45% |
| Potassium 235mg | 6% |

\* The % Daily Value (DV) tells you how much a nutrient in a serving of food contributes to a daily diet. 2,000 calories a day is used for general nutrition advice.

**Ingredients:** water, tomato purée (water, tomato paste), seasoned beef crumbles (beef, salt, spice extracts), diced tomatoes in tomato juice, red kidney beans, kidney beans. Contains less than 2% of the following ingredients: concentrate (caramel color added), jalapeno peppers, salt, dehydrated onions, **sugar,** dehydrated garlic, paprika, red pepper, soybean oil, soy lecithin, mono and diglycerides, mixed tocopherols, ascorbic acid, flavoring.

The Nutrition Facts label and ingredients list on a food label can help you with your food choices.

*Check the Serving Size.* Calorie and nutrient information on the label is for one serving of this size.

*Look at Calories per serving.* Use the calories listed to compare similar products (check to make sure the Serving Size is the same).

*Look at the grams of Total Fat in 1 serving.* To help lower your risk of heart disease, try to choose foods that are low in saturated fats, trans fats, and cholesterol.

*Check the grams of Total Carbohydrate.* This is the total amount of starches, natural and added sugars, sugar alcohols, and dietary fiber in a food. If you count carbs using carb Choices, divide the Total Carbohydrate amount by 15 to determine how many carb Choices are in one serving (1 carb choice has 15 grams of carbs).

*Look for foods that have Dietary Fiber.* A good source of fiber is about 3 grams of fiber per serving and an excellent source has at least 5 grams or more per serving.

*Choose foods that are lower in Added Sugars.* Total sugars include sugars that are naturally in foods (such as in fruit and dairy products) and sugars that are added to foods. Added Sugars tell you how much of the Total Carbohydrate amount comes from sugars added to the food. Every 4 grams of sugar is equal to 1 teaspoon. Look for food products that have little to no added sugars.

For more help using the information on food labels, ask your dietitian.

# STOCKING A DIABETES-FRIENDLY PANTRY

Having a well-stocked pantry of go-to items for cooking makes it so much easier when it comes time to meal plan, shop, and cook. Some pantry staples will cut down on shopping and prep time and save money in the long run by reducing food waste.

Must-have items in your kitchen:

- Cooking oils such as olive oil, canola oil, and nonstick cooking spray
- Condiments such as vinegars, mustard, hot sauce, lower-sodium soy sauce, light mayonnaise, and reduced-sugar ketchup and BBQ sauce. Check the Nutrition Facts label for added sugars and sodium—choose products with less sodium and little to no added sugars.
- Salad dressings are good to have on hand for making a quick salad. Bottle salad dressings can be surprisingly high in

sugar—check the Nutrition Facts label and choose dressings with little to no added sugar. (You can also try making your own salad dressing! See page 84 for recipes.)

- Spices and seasonings such as salt, ground black pepper, salt-free seasoning blends, dried herbs, garlic powder, onion powder, cinnamon, chili powder, and ground cumin
- Whole grains (see Chapter 3 on cooking methods) such as brown rice, oatmeal, hulled barley and quinoa, and whole-grain breads. When shopping for bread, look for "100% whole grain" or "100% whole wheat" on the package.
- Produce items such as onions, garlic, celery, carrots, tomato, lettuce for salads, and favorite vegetables and fruits that are in season
- Canned goods (always look for low-sodium or no-salt-added) such as broth, beans, tomatoes, tuna, chicken, salmon (look for protein packed in water not oil), and fruits packed in water or its own 100% juice (no added sugar)
- Sweeteners such as honey and sugar substitutes
- Frozen items such as frozen fruit, frozen vegetables, or frozen cuts of meat and fish
- Sunflower seeds, nuts, and nut butters (look for natural nut butters with no added sugars)

# RESOURCES TO HELP WITH GROCERIES

There are times in our lives when our budgets are tighter than others. The good news is that there are many resources available to help you get groceries when money is tight. If you need immediate access to groceries, there is a network of over 200 food banks across the U.S. that work with food pantries and meal programs to offer relief. To find your local food bank, visit Feeding America's website and use their Food Bank locator: **https://www.feedingamerica.org/find-your-local-foodbank**. You can also call Feeding America toll-free at 1-800-771-2303. Once you find your local food bank, you can reach out to them to find out more about their programs and which local food pantries and meal programs they use to help access food. Using a food bank is the best way to get food immediately.

If you don't need immediate access to food, but need help with money for groceries, you can also find out if you qualify for the Supplemental Nutrition Assistance Program (SNAP, formerly known as Food Stamps). Each state handles SNAP assistance differently, so the best place to start is with your local food bank to see if they can help you learn more about SNAP and apply for benefits. If they don't, you can search the U.S. Department of Agriculture (USDA) website to find out if you are eligible (**https://www.fns.usda.gov/snap/recipient/eligibility**) and where to apply for benefits in your state (**https://www.fns.usda.gov/snap/state-directory**). You can also call the toll-free SNAP information hotline at 1-800-221-5689.

There are many misconceptions and myths about the SNAP program. It is important for you to know that federal programs like SNAP, which currently helps 1 in 7 Americans, offer families the extra help they need to purchase nutritious food during difficult times, and you are entitled to those benefits should you need and qualify for them. Having SNAP benefits does not prohibit you from using other food resources like food banks and food pantries.

If you have children or are a senior (60 years of age or older), there are additional programs available to access food. Your local food bank will likely have resources for you to access them. If not, you can reach out to the following organizations for help:

## PROGRAMS FOR CHILDREN 18 AND UNDER:

**Food and Nutrition Service (USDA)**

https://www.fns.usda.gov/programs

## PROGRAMS FOR SENIORS AGE 60 YEARS OR OLDER:

**National Council on Aging (NCOA)**

https://www.ncoa.org/older-adults-caregivers
Or call the NCOA at 571-527-3900.

## NATIONAL HUNGER HOTLINE

**By Phone:** Call the USDA National Hunger Hotline, which operates from 7:00 AM – 10:00 PM Eastern Time. If you need food assistance, call 1-866-3-HUNGRY or 1-877-8-HAMBRE to speak with a representative who will find food resources such as meal sites, food banks, and other social services available near your location.

**By Text:** Text "97779" to the automated service with a question that may contain a keyword such as "food," "summer," "meals," to receive an automated response to resources located near an address and/or zip code.

# CHAPTER 3

## Diabetes-Friendly Meal Planning and Cooking

### THE DIABETES PLATE METHOD

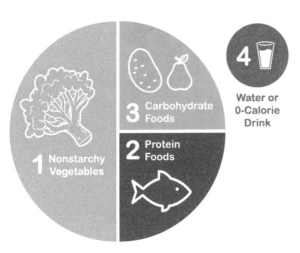

The Diabetes Plate Method is the easiest way to create healthy meals that can help manage blood glucose. Using this method, you can create perfectly portioned meals with a healthy balance of vegetables, protein, and carbohydrates—without any counting, calculating, weighing, or measuring. All you need is a plate!

To start out, you need a plate that is not too big. The size of our plate usually determines the size of our portions, so you want to start with a reasonably sized plate—we recommend about 9 inches across (about the width of a sheet of paper).

If your dinner plates are larger than this, try using a smaller salad or dessert plate for your meals. Or, if your dinner plates have a lip or artwork inside the edge, use that as a border for filling your plate.

Now that you have the right plate, it's time to fill it! Imagine two lines drawn on your plate breaking it up into three sections:

## 1. Fill half of your plate with nonstarchy vegetables.

Nonstarchy vegetables are lower in carbohydrate, so they do not raise blood glucose much. They are also high in vitamins, minerals, and fiber, making them an important part of a healthy diet. Filling half your plate with nonstarchy vegetables means you will get plenty of servings of these superfoods.

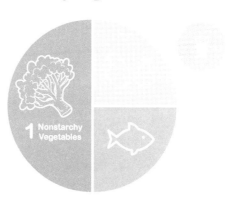

*Examples of nonstarchy vegetables include:*

- Amaranth greens or Chinese spinach
- Artichoke
- Asparagus
- Baby corn
- Bamboo shoots
- Beans (green, wax, Italian)
- Bean sprouts
- Beets
- Brussels sprouts
- Broccoli
- Cabbage (green, bok choy, Chinese)
- Carrots
- Cauliflower
- Celery
- Chayote
- Cucumber
- Daikon
- Eggplant

- Greens (collard, kale, mustard, turnip)
- Jicama
- Kohlrabi
- Leeks
- Mushrooms
- Okra
- Onions
- Pea pods
- Peppers
- Radishes
- Salad greens (chicory, endive, escarole, lettuce, romaine, spinach, arugula, radicchio, watercress)
- Sprouts
- Squash (summer, crookneck, spaghetti, zucchini)
- Sugar snap peas
- Swiss chard
- Tomatoes
- Turnips

## 2. Fill one-quarter of your plate with lean protein foods.

Foods high in protein such as fish, chicken, lean beef, soy products, and cheese are all considered "protein foods." Protein foods (especially those from animal sources) usually contain saturated fat, which may increase your risk of heart disease. Lean proteins are lower in fat and saturated fat, making them a healthier choice.

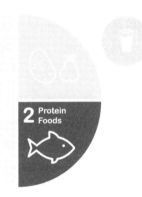

*Here are some examples of lean protein foods:*

**Animal-based**
- Chicken and turkey
- Eggs
- Fish and shellfish

- Lean beef cuts such as chuck, round, sirloin, flank, or tenderloin
- Lean pork cuts such as center loin chop or tenderloin
- Lamb
- Lean deli meats (look for low- or reduced-sodium/salt)
- Cheese and cottage cheese

**Plant-based**

- Beans
- Lentils
- Hummus and falafel
- Nuts and nut butters
- Edamame
- Tofu and tempeh
- Plant-based meat substitutes

## 3. Fill one-quarter of your plate with carbohydrate foods.

Foods that are higher in carbohydrate include grains, starchy vegetables, beans and legumes, fruit, yogurt, and milk. These foods have the greatest effect on blood glucose levels. Limiting your portion of carbohydrate foods to one-quarter of your plate can help keep blood glucose levels from 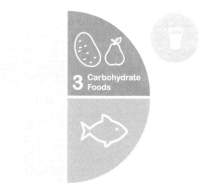 rising too high after meals. Keep in mind that some plant-based protein foods (like beans and legumes) are also high in carbohydrates.

*Here are some examples of carbohydrate foods:*

**Grains**

- Brown rice
- Bulgur
- Grits
- Oatmeal
- Polenta
- Popcorn

- Quinoa
- Sorghum
- Grain products such as bread, pasta, and tortillas

## Starchy vegetables

- Acorn squash
- Butternut squash
- Corn
- Green peas
- Parsnips
- Plantain
- Potato
- Pumpkin
- Sweet potato/yam

## Beans and legumes

- Beans such as black, pinto, and kidney
- Baked beans
- Chickpeas/ garbanzo beans and hummus
- Lentils
- Refried beans

## Fruits

- Apples and applesauce
- Bananas
- Berries
- Cherries
- Dried fruit
- Grapefruit
- Kiwi
- Mango
- Melons (all types)
- Oranges
- Papaya
- Peaches
- Pears
- Pineapple
- Plums

## Dairy

- Low-fat or fat-free milk
- Plain soy milk
- Yogurt

## 4. Choose water or a low-calorie drink.

Water is the best choice because
it contains no calories or carbohydrates and has no effect on blood
glucose. Other zero- or low-calorie
drink options include:

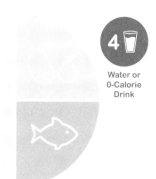

Water or
0-Calorie
Drink

- Unsweetened tea (hot or
  iced)
- Unsweetened coffee (hot
  or iced)
- Sparkling water/club soda, plain or flavored without added sugar.
- Flavored or infused water made without added sugar
- Diet soda or other diet drinks

## WHAT ABOUT COMBINATION FOODS?

Our meals don't always fit neatly into the sections of the plate. Many
dishes combine the different food types together, such as soups, casseroles, sandwiches, pizza, or pasta.

You can still use the plate method when preparing and portioning combination foods. Just identify the different foods in the dish and think about
where they would fit in the plate.

For example, in a slice of pizza, the crust would be the carbohydrate
food, the cheese and any meats on top would be the protein foods, and
the tomato sauce and any vegetables on top would be the nonstarchy
vegetables.

Try to prepare combination dishes with the same proportions as the plate.
So, to build a pizza using the plate method, choose thin crust to reduce
the portion of carbohydrates and top it with lots of vegetables instead of

meat (or choose a lean meat). Stick to just one or two slices and serve with a side salad so that half your meal is nonstarchy vegetables.

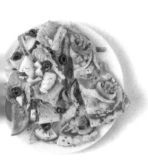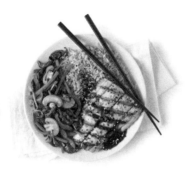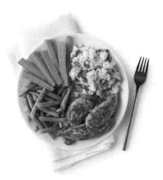

# HEALTHY COOKING TIPS

Healthy cooking can seem intimidating because we often equate "healthy" with lacking variety or flavor. Nothing could be further from the truth! Healthy cooking provides you with a great variety of food types, tastes, and textures. Knowing how to maximize those attributes of your ingredients with these easy tips will make healthy cooking all that more appealing.

## SUBSTITUTE STARCHES WITH VEGETABLES

Wherever you can, substitute all or some of your starch options with vegetables. Thankfully, vegetables are so versatile, it's easy to do. There are products on the market that make this swap easy, and there are kitchen tools that can help, too.

- *Spiralized zucchini, summer squash or other vegetables.* Eat raw or steam for a few minutes until tender. Use in place of spaghetti noodles. Buy already spiralized produce in a bag from the produce or freezer sections of the grocery store. Or buy a spiralizer and make your own at home. You can also spiralize starchier vegetables like sweet potatoes, butternut squash, and potatoes.

*Cauliflower rice.* Buy in a bag in the produce section or the freezer section. Make your own by processing a whole head of cauliflower in the food proces-

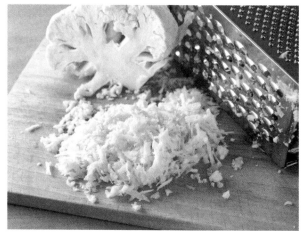

sor until cut up into small, rice-size pieces, or grate cauliflower using a box grater. Steam until cooked through and substitute for rice, barley, quinoa, or other grains in any recipe.

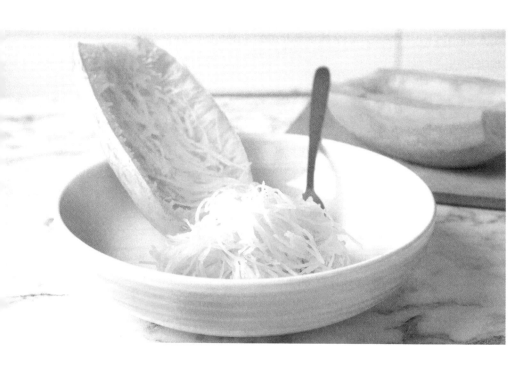

■ *Spaghetti squash.* Nature took care of this one for you. Simply cook, de-seed, and pull the squash flesh out of the skin and use just like angel hair pasta (see Basic Spaghetti Squash on page 81).

**Ways to cut down on carbohydrates:**

| Ingredient | Healthier swap |
| --- | --- |
| Sugar in baking | Use 30%–50% less sugar or a baking sugar blend. |
| Sugar added to coffee, tea, or other drinks | Use a sugar substitute. |
| Breadcrumbs | Ground nuts |
| Spaghetti | Spaghetti squash or spiralized zucchini ("zoodles") |
| Rice | Make cauliflower rice by grating or finely chopping cauliflower florets (cauliflower rice is also available in many groceries stores in the produce section or with frozen vegetables). |
| Hash browns | Grated zucchini or yellow squash |
| Mashed potatoes | Replace half or more of potatoes with cauliflower. |
| Pizza crust | Try thin, flatbread, or cauliflower pizza crust or use portobello mushroom caps instead of bread. |
| Sandwich bread or wrap | Wrap filling in leaf lettuce or cabbage leaves, or use one slice of bread for an "open-face" sandwich. |
| Flour tortillas | Use corn tortillas or high-fiber, low-carb tortillas such as those made by La Tortilla Factory. |
| Pasta dishes | Use less pasta per serving and bulk up the dish with nonstarchy vegetables such as broccoli, mushrooms, spinach, tomatoes, zucchini, and others, or substitute pasta for a different whole grain such as brown rice, barley, oatmeal, or quinoa. |

## Ways to increase fiber:

| Ingredient | Healthier swap |
| --- | --- |
| All-purpose flour | Whole-wheat flour |
| Regular pasta | Whole-wheat pasta or pasta made from beans/legumes, such as lentil pasta, or substitute pasta for a different whole grain such as brown rice, barley, oatmeal, or quinoa |
| White rice | Brown rice or other whole grain such as quinoa or barley |
| Breadcrumbs | Chopped oats or almond meal |
| White bread | Whole-grain bread (look for "100% whole grain" on the package) |
| Ground beef | Replace half of the beef with lentils or beans such as black, pinto, kidney, or white beans. |

## Ways to reduce calories and fat in recipes:

| Ingredient | Healthier swap |
| --- | --- |
| Butter or oil to sauté | Use olive oil– or canola oil–based nonstick cooking spray. |
| Butter or shortening in baking | Replace half with unsweetened applesauce. |
| Heavy cream | Replace with evaporated skim milk. |
| Whole milk | Replace with 2%, 1%, or nonfat milk. |
| Sour cream | Use reduced-fat sour cream or fat-free, plain Greek yogurt. |
| Regular cheese | Use less (use stronger-flavored cheese—a little bit goes a long way) or try reduced-fat cheese. |
| Cream cheese | Reduced-fat or light cream cheese, fat-free ricotta cheese |
| Bacon | Canadian bacon, vegetarian bacon, turkey bacon, or vegetarian bacon bits |
| Ground beef | Extra-lean ground beef (ground sirloin), lean ground chicken or turkey, or swap some ground meat for beans |
| Hamburger | Use lean ground beef or ground chicken or turkey. Add chopped mushrooms, shredded zucchini, and/or chopped onions to add bulk. |
| Mayonnaise | Light mayonnaise or fat-free, plain Greek yogurt |

## Ways to reduce sodium/salt:

| Ingredient | Healthier swap |
| --- | --- |
| Salt in recipes | Add less salt than instructed when cooking. If possible, taste before adding salt. Use fresh or dried herbs and spices or salt-free seasonings for flavor. |
| Salt on vegetables | Fresh-squeezed lemon or vinegar |
| Soy sauce | Use reduced-sodium or lower-sodium versions. |
| Broth | Use reduced-sodium, low-sodium, or no-salt-added versions. |
| Canned vegetables and beans | Use reduced-sodium, low-sodium, or no-salt-added versions. Drain and rinse before using. |
| Ground beef | Replace half of the beef with lentils or beans such as black, pinto, kidney, or white beans. |

# CHAPTER 4

# Easy Prepping and Storage

Once you've made your plan for what you will eat for the week, you can set yourself up for easy prepping. Here are some guidelines on how to make the most out of your meal preparation.

1.  Read the recipes you are using and make a list of all ingredients and equipment you will need, noting amounts. Make a list separating your ingredients by category. Here is an example:

| Protein | Produce | Dairy | Dry | Freezer | Other |
|---------|---------|-------|-----|---------|-------|
| 90% lean ground beef, 1 pound | 1 head of broccoli | 8 ounces fat-free, plain Greek yogurt | 15-ounce can no-salt-added diced tomatoes ×2 | 12-ounce bag steamable cauliflower rice | Quart-size freezer bags |

2.  After making your list, but before shopping, clean out your refrigerator. Check if there are any staple items that are running low and add them to your list. Using your grocery list and recipes, check to see what items you already have on hand, and make sure they are still good and that you have enough for the meals you are planning to make.

3.  Do the dishes and clean the counters. Your kitchen will be clean and ready for you to dive in to your food prepping.

4.  Set yourself up to prep:

    *   Empty the dishwasher so you can clean as you go.

- Get out your cutting board, knives, and the rest of the utensils you'll need to prep.
- Set out a "garbage bowl," which is a big bowl you set on your counter to throw scraps and packaging in so you don't have to keep running back and forth to the garbage can. This step keeps your food prep–area clean.
- Read your recipe all the way through again so you know if there are any precooking steps you need to take such as preheating an oven.
- Gather your ingredients, equipment, and your food storage containers.

5. Start prepping and cooking!

# MEAL PREP TIPS

There are many strategies for meal prep and planning. One way to approach meal prep is to prepare several recipes all at once, then portion meals into individual containers to reheat throughout the week. For example, on a day when you have time to spend a couple hours in the kitchen, you could prepare a few different entrée and side recipes to eat throughout the week. For perfectly portioned meals that can be taken to go, portion out the entrees and sides into individual meals in airtight to-go containers. This strategy is great for preparing lunches to take to work, or having single-serving dinners ready to reheat on busy weeknights.

Another strategy is to prepare ingredients ahead of time to cut down on prep time when you are cooking a meal. For example, here are some ingredients that could be prepared ahead of time for meals later in the week:

1. *Cook protein* (For example, lean ground beef or turkey [see recipe on page 102] and shredded chicken [see recipes on page 95–100]). You can leave the meat unseasoned for now and add seasoning to it when you are ready to use it. That way, you aren't stuck with a pound of taco meat if you don't feel like tacos later in the week. Now you can use the cooked meat for a quick skillet meal or mix it with marinara sauce for spaghetti.

2. *Cut up veggies* (Use raw veggies for salads and dipping [see recipe on page 75] and roasted vegetables for everything else [see recipe on page 78]). Store your cut, raw veggies in airtight containers in the refrigerator for up to 1 week. If they are looking dry at the end of the week, rinse them in cold water and pat dry to refresh them.

3. *Cut up fruit* Portion in freezer bags for smoothies (see recipe on page 117).

4. *Cook your basic starches* Try the following foods:
   - Brown rice (see recipe on page 59)
   - Oatmeal (see recipe on page 61)
   - Quinoa (see recipe on page 66)
   - Barley (see recipe on page 68)
   - Sweet potatoes (see recipe on page 83)

5. *Portion out your snacks* This helps prevent you from overeating them out of the box, bag, or bowl.

With these ingredients prepped, you can quickly throw together a satisfying meal in minutes. See the section on

**CHEF TIP**

If you are storing items in the freezer, label and date them so you know how long they've been in there.

"Throw-It-Together Meals" (page 112) for recipes ideas using prepared ingredients.

# PRODUCE PREP AND STORAGE

Prepping produce ahead of time can be a great time-saver in the long run. Investing a little bit of time at the beginning of the week to stock your refrigerator with cleaned, cut-up vegetables and fruits will make you more likely to eat them than if they aren't prepped and ready to eat. Making them easy to grab and go will help you raise your vegetable and fruit intake every day.

Prepping vegetables ahead of time can also be a helpful shortcut when preparing meals on a busy weeknight.

Follow these simple steps to set yourself up for success:

1. Washing
   - Wash vegetables and fruits that you plan on immediately cutting and storing so they are ready to eat at a moment's notice. Examples of these vegetables are cucumbers, broccoli, carrots, bell peppers, and cauliflower. Wait to wash whole produce that you won't cut up until it's time to cook, especially delicate items such as fresh herbs and berries. These types of produce will go bad faster if you wash them too far ahead of time.
   - When washing certain items, you want to do a thorough job to avoid any food safety issues but also preserve the integrity of the ingredient.
     - Wipe mushrooms with a damp towel to remove all dirt, but do not rinse or submerge in water. Using water will make them spongy.

- Thoroughly wash and dry lettuces, ideally using a salad spinner if you have one. If you don't, dry the leaves with a paper towel.
- Scrub potatoes with a dedicated vegetable scrubber or a clean kitchen towel and running water. If baking the potatoes, dry them well before putting in the oven. If peeling the potatoes, rinse them again after peeling.
- Wash items that have skin you will cut through, such as melons, avocados, lemons, limes, and oranges.
- Produce such as broccoli, cauliflower, and kale should be soaked in cold water for a few minutes before washing to loosen any dirt that might be stuck in the crevices.

2. Prepping

- Once your produce is clean and ready to be prepped, keep it in a bowl and 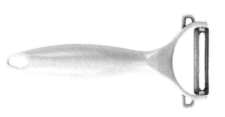 ensure your cutting board, peeler, and knife are clean. Have food storage or prep bowls ready for the cut produce, and if you are not going straight to cooking from prepping, store all cut produce immediately in the refrigerator or freezer (if prepping to freeze, see below).

- Peels can be left on most produce if it has been cleaned properly. Unless a recipe calls for peeling, there is no need to peel cucumber, potatoes, carrots, zucchini, yellow squash, or sweet potatoes. Onions, garlic, pineapples, avocados, bananas, citrus fruits, and melons should be peeled before eating or cooking.

- Search YouTube for videos on the best ways to cut various kinds of produce. Channels such as America's Test Kitchen, Epicurious, Food52, and Tastemade offer excellent introductory and more advanced knife-skill videos.

3. Storing

- To refrigerate or not? That is the question. It is important to store produce properly to maintain freshness and quality. Here is a list of produce to store in the refrigerator and a list of produce to store on the counter or in a cabinet:
- Refrigerator:

  - All cut produce (usually good for up to 1 week in an airtight container)
  - Lettuce and salad greens (wrap in a damp paper towel to maintain crispness)

## CHEF TIP

Refrigerating tomatoes is not recommended because it can affect their flavor and texture. But, if you have overripe tomatoes that you are not using soon, storing them in the fridge will prevent rotting for a few more days. Use these tomatoes for cooked dishes like pasta sauce instead of eating raw in salads.

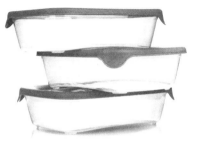

- Fresh herbs (except fresh basil; put basil in a vase with water, like you would for flowers, and place on the counter or window sill)
- Cucumbers
- Bell peppers
- Broccoli and cauliflower
- Celery
- Carrots
- Green beans
- Asparagus (store in a glass or jar with the stems in an inch or two of water)
- Zucchini and summer squash
- Apples
- Citrus fruits (oranges, lemons, limes, grapefruit)
- Grapes
- Berries

- Counter or cabinet:
  - Onions (always store away from all other produce)
  - Garlic
  - Bananas
  - Avocados until ripe, and then refrigerate to extend shelf life
  - Tomatoes (see Chef Tip on previous page)
  - Potatoes and sweet potatoes
  - Winter squash
  - Melons

4. Freezing

- Freezing produce is a great way to extend its shelf life and to maximize your budget by buying certain produce in season, when it is more budget friendly. However, not all produce freezes the same, and you may destroy the ingredient if it isn't frozen properly. Some items can be frozen from raw and some need further cooking or processing:

- Freeze raw:

  - Fruit: Whole or pitted berries and cherries, peeled and cut pineapple, mango, bananas, avocado, and melon. When thawed, these fruits will not have them same fresh texture as when they were raw. Use them in cooking or smoothies for best results.

  - Vegetables and herbs: Cut bell peppers, peeled and cut onions, cut zucchini, cut summer squash, peeled and cut winter squash, asparagus, green beans, kale, and fresh herbs. When thawed, these vegetables will not have the same fresh texture as when they were raw. Use them in cooking or smoothies for best results.

## HOW TO FREEZE PRODUCE PROPERLY

Wash, peel (if needed), and chop into bite-sized pieces (or leave whole for small items like berries), and then lay the item out on a baking sheet and freeze until solid (at least 2 hours). Once frozen, transfer to a freezer-safe bag or other freezer container. Store up to 6 months in the freezer. You can also freeze diced vegetables such as onion, bell peppers, carrots, and celery to cut down on prep time. Simply dice the produce and store in pre-portioned, freezer-safe bags or other containers.

## HOW TO FREEZE COOKED OR PAR-COOKED PRODUCE

Any cooked items like roasted vegetables, apples, and pears should be cooled and can be stored in a freezer bag or other freezer-safe container for up to 6 months.

Some raw vegetables should be par-cooked or blanched before freezing. Blanching involves slightly cooking raw produce in boiling water for as little as one minute, then plunging into ice water to stop the cooking. This process results in frozen produce with better color, texture, and flavor.

Fruits and vegetables that should be cooked or par-cooked (blanched) before freezing:

*Fruits:* Apples, pears

*Vegetables:* Carrots, celery, tomatoes, eggplant, spaghetti squash, potatoes, sweet potatoes, broccoli, cauliflower, spinach

How to blanch fruits and vegetables for freezing:

1.  Bring a pot of water to a boil. While waiting for the water to boil, prepare a bowl of ice water and a baking sheet lined with a clean kitchen towel or paper towels.
2.  Drop the ingredient into the boiling water for 1 minute, remove from the boiling water, and immediately submerge in the ice water.
3.  Remove from the ice water, place onto the clean towel, and pat or squeeze dry.
4.  Place into a freezer bag or other freezer-safe container and store in the freezer for up to 6 months.

# STORING AND REHEATING LEFTOVERS

## HOW TO STORE LEFTOVERS SAFELY

After cooking your diabetic-friendly meals, leftovers can be stored in the refrigerator for up to 6 days, or you can freeze the food. Protein dishes can be frozen for 3–4 months, and non-protein dishes can be frozen for 6 months. Store in airtight containers (make sure they are freezer safe if you plan to store in the freezer).

A good strategy for storing leftovers is to store individual servings in separate containers. This way, you have properly portioned meals ready to go, and you won't have to thaw or reheat more food than you plan on eating.

## HOW TO THAW LEFTOVERS SAFELY

When thawing leftovers, you can do so safely by putting them in the refrigerator, in cold water, and in the microwave oven. Refrigerator thawing takes the longest, but your leftovers stay safe the whole time. After thawing, the food should be used within 3–4 days or can be refrozen.

If you choose to use cold water to thaw your food, it is faster than thawing in the refrigerator, but requires more attention. The frozen leftovers must be in a leak-proof package or plastic bag. If the bag leaks, water can get into the food, and bacteria from the air or surrounding environment could enter the bag. Foods thawed by cold water should be cooked before refreezing.

If you need to thaw the food quickly, microwaving is the fastest method. In the microwave, heat the frozen food until it reaches 165°F. You can measure the temperature with a food thermometer. After heating the food to this temperature, it is safe to refreeze.

## REHEATING LEFTOVERS WITHOUT THAWING

Using either a saucepan (in the case of a soup or stew) or the oven or microwave (for example, for casseroles and combination meals), it is safe to reheat frozen leftovers without thawing. This reheating process will take longer than if the food is thawed first, but this option is safe for when time is short to make a meal.

## HOW TO REHEAT LEFTOVERS SAFELY

If leftovers are not stored in individual serving containers, portion out one serving to reheat, instead of reheating the whole batch. Repeatedly reheating and chilling leftovers can cause more bacteria growth, so only reheat what you plan to eat at that time.

Food Safety Tip: To keep leftover foods safe, you want to keep them out of the "Danger Zone" (40°F–140°F) where bacteria grow easily. Storing foods below 40°F (in the refrigerator) prevents bacteria growth, and heating leftovers to at least 165°F kills bacteria.

Every time you chill and reheat leftover foods, they are spending time in the Danger Zone, so you should avoid chilling and reheating leftovers more than one or two times. Instead of reheating large batches of leftovers, store leftovers in individual servings, or portion out one serving from the fridge, and only reheat what you need for that meal.

Thawing food in the fridge and then refreezing is safe because the food has been kept below 40°F the whole time. However, you should avoid thawing and refreezing foods too many times because it can affect the texture and flavor.

Make sure foods reach 165°F on a food thermometer when reheating leftovers. If reheating sauces, soups, and gravies, bring them to a rolling boil. Covering the leftovers while reheating helps retain moisture and makes sure that the food heats all the way through.

When reheating food in the microwave, make sure to cover and rotate the food so it heats evenly. Evenly place the food in a covered microwave-safe ceramic or glass dish, and add a little liquid if needed. Vent the lid of the microwave-safe container or cover with a paper towel to let the steam escape. Creating moist heat helps destroy harmful bacteria and ensures uniform cooking. Microwaves have cold spots, so make sure to check the temperature of the food in several places with a food thermometer. Also, allow the food to rest before checking the internal temperature. Cooking continues for a longer time in dense foods like a beef roast or whole turkey than in less dense foods like fruits, small vegetables, and breads.

## HOW TO PROPERLY REFREEZE PREVIOUSLY FROZEN LEFTOVERS

Sometimes there are "leftover leftovers." If you have cooked your previously frozen leftovers to the safe temperature of 165°F, it is safe to refreeze any food remaining. Make sure you always use a food thermometer to measure the food temperature properly. If you have a large container of frozen leftovers, you can thaw the container in the refrigerator, take out the portion you wish to heat, and safely refreeze the rest of the unheated portion.

Information adapted from U.S. Department of Agriculture Food Safety and Inspection Service. Find more information on food safety here: https://www.fsis.usda.gov/wps/portal/fsis/topics/food-safety-education/get-answers/food-safety-fact-sheets/safe-food-handling/leftovers-and-food-safety/ct_index

# CHAPTER 5

## Recipes

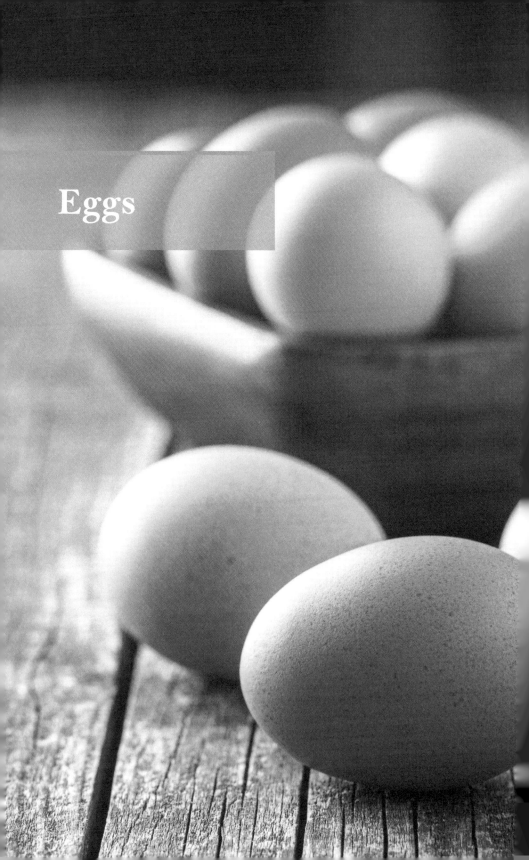

# Eggs

# Hard-Boiled Eggs

SERVES 6 ■ SERVING SIZE 1 egg
PREP TIME 2 minutes ■ COOK TIME 20 minutes

6 large eggs
Water

## CHEF TIP

Buy and refrigerate the eggs you plan to hard boil 10 days to 2 weeks before you hard boil them. Older eggs hard boil and peel better than fresh eggs. Also, if you overcook them, the yolk will get a greenish ring around it. It's perfectly fine to eat; that just means the egg is slightly overcooked.

## WAYS TO USE

- Deviled Eggs
  (see page 52)
- Easy Egg Salad
  (see page 53)
- Eggs on toast: Chop up eggs, season with 1/4 teaspoon salt and 1/4 teaspoon pepper, and serve on whole-grain toast. Additional toppings can include salsa, guacamole, hummus, fresh herbs, Roasted Vegetables (see page 78), or cheese.

1 Lay the eggs in a single layer on the bottom of a large saucepan and cover with cold water so that there is about 1 inch of water over the eggs.

2 Place the pan on a stovetop burner, but before turning on the heat, set a timer for 20 minutes.

3 Start the timer, turn the heat to high, and bring to a boil. Once boiling, reduce to a gentle simmer and simmer until the timer goes off. Meanwhile, prepare a bowl of ice water.

4 When the timer goes off, immediately drain the water from the pan, and then gently shake the eggs in the pan to crack the shells.

5 Cover the eggs with the ice water and let sit for 15 minutes.

6 Drain the ice water, gently roll each egg on a paper towel to loosen the shell, and peel the shell off.

7 Store in an airtight container in the refrigerator for up to 1 week.

### Choices/Exchanges
1 Medium-Fat Protein

### Basic Nutritional Values

| | | | |
|---|---|---|---|
| **Calories** | 80 | **Potassium** | 65 mg |
| Calories from Fat | 45 | **Total Carbohydrate** | 1 g |
| **Total Fat** | 5.5 g | Dietary Fiber | 0 g |
| Saturated Fat | 1.6 g | Sugars | 1 g |
| Trans Fat | 0 g | Added Sugars | 0 g |
| **Cholesterol** | 185 mg | **Protein** | 6 g |
| **Sodium** | 60 mg | **Phosphorus** | 85 mg |

# Deviled Eggs

SERVES 6 ■ SERVING SIZE 2 stuffed egg halves
PREP TIME 5 minutes ■ COOK TIME 0 minutes

6 large hard-boiled eggs, peeled and cooled (see previous recipe)

1/4 cup fat-free, plain Greek yogurt

2 Tablespoons salsa

1/4 teaspoon salt

1/4 teaspoon ground black pepper

**Optional ingredients:**

1/2 teaspoon chili powder

1 Tablespoon finely chopped cilantro or parsley

1 Cut the eggs in half lengthwise (vertically) and scoop the yolks out into a small bowl. Mash with a fork.

2 Add the yogurt, salsa, salt, and pepper and mix to combine.

3 Using a spoon, evenly distribute the filling into each egg half.

4 Optional: Sprinkle 1/2 teaspoon chili powder and 1 Tablespoon finely chopped cilantro or parsley evenly over the top of the egg halves.

## CHEF TIP

You can replace the salsa with 2 teaspoons Dijon mustard to make a more traditional deviled egg. Top with a sprinkle of paprika or dried dill.

**Choices/Exchanges**
1 Medium-Fat Protein

**Basic Nutritional Values**

| | |
|---|---|
| **Calories** | 80 |
| Calories from Fat | 45 |
| **Total Fat** | 5.0 g |
| Saturated Fat | 1.7 g |
| Trans Fat | 0.0 g |
| **Cholesterol** | 185 mg |
| **Sodium** | 190 mg |
| **Potassium** | 95 mg |
| **Total Carbohydrate** | 1 g |
| Dietary Fiber | 0 g |
| Sugars | 1 g |
| Added Sugars | 0 g |
| **Protein** | 7 g |
| **Phosphorus** | 105 mg |

# Easy Egg Salad

SERVES 6 ■ SERVING SIZE 1/3 cup
PREP TIME 5 minutes ■ COOK TIME 20 minutes

6 large hard-boiled eggs, cooled and peeled

1 rib of celery, small dice

1/4 cup light mayonnaise

1 teaspoon Dijon mustard

1/4 teaspoon ground black pepper

1 Cut hard-boiled eggs in half and remove and discard half of the egg yolks (you should end up with 6 whole egg whites and 3 whole egg yolks total). Add to a medium bowl and lightly mash with a fork.

2 Add the remaining ingredients and stir to combine.

3 Store in an airtight container in the refrigerator for up to 1 week.

## CHEF TIP

Serve the egg salad on a bed of salad greens, on whole-grain toast, in a whole-grain tortilla wrap, on whole-grain crackers, or with whole-grain tortilla chips.

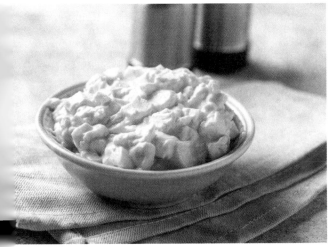

**Choices/Exchanges**
1 Lean Protein, 1/2 Fat

**Basic Nutritional Values**

| | |
|---|---|
| **Calories** | 70 |
| Calories from Fat | 40 |
| **Total Fat** | 4.5 g |
| Saturated Fat | 1.0 g |
| Trans Fat | 0.0 g |
| **Cholesterol** | 90 mg |
| **Sodium** | 150 mg |
| **Potassium** | 90 mg |
| **Total Carbohydrate** | 2 g |
| Dietary Fiber | 0 g |
| Sugars | 1 g |
| Added Sugars | 0 g |
| **Protein** | 5 g |
| **Phosphorus** | 40 mg |

# Scrambled Eggs

SERVES 6 ■ SERVING SIZE 1/2 cup
PREP TIME 5 minutes ■ COOK TIME 10 minutes

2 large eggs

2 large egg whites

2 Tablespoons fat-free, plain
   Greek yogurt

1/8 teaspoon salt

Pinch of ground black pepper

1 teaspoon olive oil

1 In a medium bowl, whisk together the whole eggs, egg whites, yogurt, salt, and pepper.

2 Add the olive oil to a nonstick skillet over medium heat.

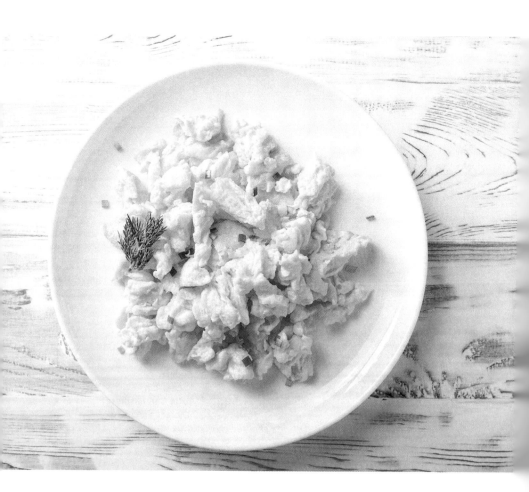

3 Pour the egg mixture into the pan and, with a heat-proof rubber spatula, scrape the bottom of the pan slowly continuously until the eggs are set and not runny. Remove from heat immediately and serve.

## COOKING SAFETY TIP

Be sure to wash your hands and food-contact surfaces when handling raw eggs. Consuming raw or undercooked meats, poultry, seafood, shellfish, or eggs may increase your risk of foodborne illness. Having raw egg on your hand or food contact surface may contaminate other food items that will not be cooked further.

## WAYS TO USE

- Serve on top of whole-grain toast and top with optional ingredients including salsa, guacamole, Roasted Vegetables (see page 78), fresh herbs, or cheese.
- Use instead of meat in a burrito, taco, quesadilla, or wrap.
- Make your own breakfast sandwich with a whole-grain English muffin, turkey bacon or sausage, and cheese.
- Stir into Brown Rice (see page 59) with Roasted Vegetables.

**Choices/Exchanges**
2 Lean Protein, 1/2 Fat

**Basic Nutritional Values**

| | |
|---|---|
| **Calories** | 120 |
| Calories from Fat | 60 |
| **Total Fat** | 7.0 g |
| Saturated Fat | 1.9 g |
| Trans Fat | 0.0 g |
| **Cholesterol** | 185 mg |
| **Sodium** | 280 mg |
| **Potassium** | 140 mg |
| **Total Carbohydrate** | 1 g |
| Dietary Fiber | 0 g |
| Sugars | 1 g |
| Added Sugars | 0 g |
| **Protein** | 11 g |
| **Phosphorus** | 125 mg |

# Egg Muffins

SERVES 12 ▪ SERVING SIZE 1 muffin
PREP TIME 10 minutes ▪ COOK TIME 25 minutes

Nonstick cooking spray

1 cup frozen, chopped, thawed and squeezed spinach, divided

6 eggs

4 egg whites

1/4 cup fat-free, plain Greek yogurt

1/4 teaspoon salt

1/4 teaspoon ground black pepper

1/4 cup grated Parmesan cheese, divided

1 Preheat the oven to 350°F.

2 Spray each cup of a 12-cup muffin pan with one spray of nonstick cooking spray.

3 Add 1 Tablespoon of the thawed spinach to the bottom of each muffin cup.

4 In a medium bowl, whisk together the eggs, egg whites, yogurt, salt, and pepper. Evenly divide the egg mixture among the 12 muffin cups.

5 Top each egg muffin with 1 teaspoon Parmesan cheese.

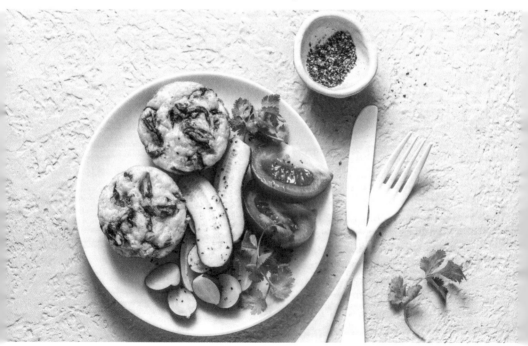

- Make a breakfast sand-wich with a toasted, whole-grain English muffin.
- Cut the muffin in half and use as a filling in a wrap or breakfast burrito.
- Serve the muffin on top of a bed of lettuce.

6 Place the muffin pan in the oven and bake for 20–25 minutes or until the eggs are slightly firm to touch.

7 Remove the pan from the oven and set aside to cool for 5 minutes.

8 Remove the muffins from the pan and serve or store in an airtight container in the refrigerator for up to 1 week.

9 To reheat from the refrigerator, place the muffin, uncovered, on a plate in the microwave and heat for 30 seconds.

## CHEF TIP

You can also store the muffins in the freezer for up to 3 months. Remove cooled muffins from the pan and arrange them on a sheet pan or plate so that they are not touching. Freeze until frozen solid, at least 2 hours, then transfer to a freezer-safe bag, or wrap individually in plastic wrap and foil. To reheat from frozen, place the muffin, uncovered, on a plate in the microwave and heat for 1 minute.

**Choices/Exchanges**
1 Lean Protein

**Basic Nutritional Values**

| | | |
|---|---|---|
| **Calories** | 50 | |
| Calories from Fat | 25 | |
| **Total Fat** | 3.0 | g |
| Saturated Fat | 1.0 | g |
| Trans Fat | 0.0 | g |
| **Cholesterol** | 95 | mg |
| **Sodium** | 135 | mg |
| **Potassium** | 105 | mg |
| **Total Carbohydrate** | 1 | g |
| Dietary Fiber | 0 | g |
| Sugars | 0 | g |
| Added Sugars | 0 | g |
| **Protein** | 6 | g |
| **Phosphorus** | 75 | mg |

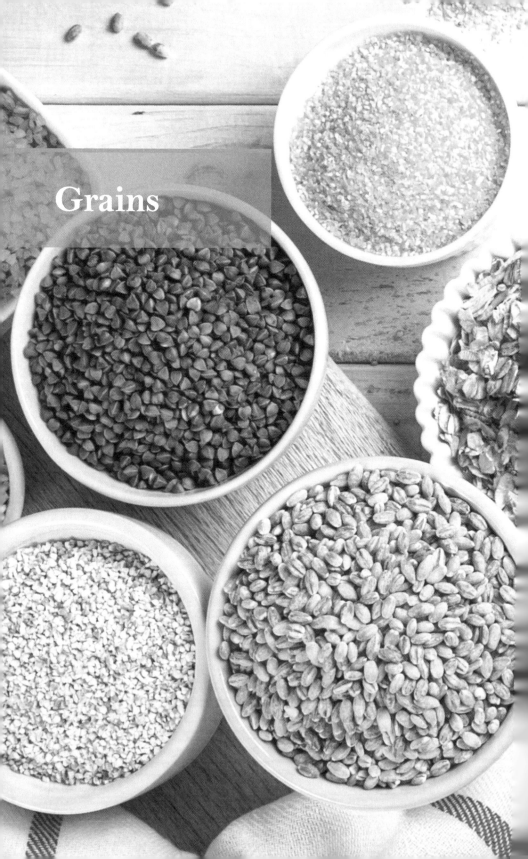

# Grains

# Brown Rice

SERVES 20 ■ SERVING SIZE 1/2 cup cooked
PREP TIME 5 minutes ■ COOK TIME 55 minutes

1 pound (16 ounces) long-grain brown rice (not instant)

5 cups water

1 Add the brown rice and 5 cups of cold water to a stock pot and cook over high heat.

2 Bring to a boil and then reduce to a simmer.

3 Cover and simmer for 45 minutes. Do not lift the lid during cooking, or you will release the steam and the rice will take longer to cook and become mushy.

4 After the 45 minutes, keep the rice covered and remove from the heat for 10 minutes.

5 Remove the lid and fluff the rice with a fork.

6 This rice can be used in any recipe calling for cooked brown rice.

7 Store in an airtight container in the refrigerator for up to 1 week, or put 1-cup portions in freezer bags and store for up to 6 months.

## WAYS TO USE

- Use as a starch side dish for any meat and vegetable.
- Mix with Scrambled Eggs (see page 54) and Roasted Vegetables (see page 78) and a dash of lower-sodium soy sauce for unfried fried rice.
- Make a burrito bowl by layering brown rice with taco meat, lettuce, salsa, and guacamole in a bowl or Mason jar.
- Use as a base for Chicken and Veggie Stir-Fry (see page 98).
- Make huevos rancheros with a serving of brown rice mixed with a serving of Scrambled Eggs (see page 54), salsa, and one spicy chicken sausage link chopped up and mixed in.
- Use to make Brown Rice Pudding (see page 60).

**Choices/Exchanges**
1 1/2 Starch

**Basic Nutritional Values**

| | | | |
|---|---|---|---|
| **Calories** | 120 | **Potassium** | 85 mg |
| Calories from Fat | 8 | **Total Carbohydrate** | 25 g |
| **Total Fat** | 1.0 g | Dietary Fiber | 2 g |
| Saturated Fat | 0.2 g | Sugars | 0 g |
| Trans Fat | 0 g | Added Sugars | 0 g |
| **Cholesterol** | 0 mg | **Protein** | 3 g |
| **Sodium** | 10 mg | **Phosphorus** | 100 mg |

# Brown Rice Pudding

SERVES 6 ■ SERVING SIZE 1/3 cup
PREP TIME 5 minutes ■ COOK TIME 10 minutes

1 cup cold 1% low-fat milk or unsweetened milk substitute such as almond or soy milk

1 teaspoon cornstarch

1 Tablespoon honey or granulated sugar substitute such as Stevia

1 1/2 teaspoons ground cinnamon, plus extra for dusting

1 teaspoon vanilla extract

1/4 teaspoon salt

2 cups cooked brown rice

1/4 cup toasted slivered almonds

1 In a saucepan off the heat, whisk together the cold milk and cornstarch until cornstarch is dissolved. Whisk in the honey, cinnamon, vanilla extract, and salt.

2 Place on the stovetop over medium-high heat. While continuing to gently whisk, bring the milk mixture to a gentle boil, and then reduce to simmer.

3 Simmer for 2 minutes. Then, using a spoon, stir in the brown rice. Continue to simmer until rice is heated through, about 5 minutes.

4 Serve warm or cold topped with the toasted slivered almonds and a sprinkle of cinnamon.

## CHEF TIP

You can change the toppings on this sweet treat by using ingredients such as any toasted nut, toasted coconut, dried fruit, sunflower or pumpkin seeds, chia seeds, or low-sugar granola.

**Choices/Exchanges**
1 Starch, 1/2 Carbohydrate, 1/2 Fat

**Basic Nutritional Values**

| | |
|---|---|
| **Calories** | 140 |
| Calories from Fat | 30 |
| **Total Fat** | 3.5 g |
| Saturated Fat | 0.6 g |
| Trans Fat | 0.0 g |
| **Cholesterol** | 4 mg |
| **Sodium** | 120 mg |
| **Potassium** | 160 mg |
| **Total Carbohydrate** | 24 g |
| Dietary Fiber | 2 g |
| Sugars | 5 g |
| Added Sugars | 3 g |
| **Protein** | 4 g |
| **Phosphorus** | 130 mg |

# Basic Oatmeal

SERVING SIZE  1/2 cup cooked oatmeal
(old-fashioned, steel-cut, or instant)

There are three main varieties of oatmeal—old-fashioned rolled oats, steel cut oats, and quick-cooking or instant oats. The different varieties require different amounts of liquid and time to cook, but the nutrition information for all three is roughly the same. The following recipes are basic cooking instructions for each type of oat, plus ideas of how to use them.

### STEEL CUT OATS

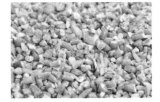

Steel cuts are whole oat grains that have been cut into smaller pieces. They take the longest to cook and produce an oatmeal with a chewy texture and rich flavor.

### OLD-FASHIONED ROLLED OATS

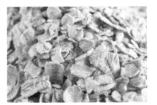

Rolled oats are whole oats that have been flattened, breaking up the hard, outer bran. They cook much faster than steel cut oats, and produce an oatmeal that is creamier, but still has a little bit of chewiness.

### QUICK-COOKING OATS

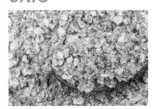

Quick-cooking or "instant" oatmeal is rolled even thinner than old-fashioned oats and cut into smaller pieces, so it cooks very quickly. The oatmeal produced by quick-cooking oats will be very creamy.

**Choices/Exchanges**
1 Starch

**Basic Nutritional Values**

| | | | |
|---|---|---|---|
| **Calories** | 85 | **Potassium** | 160 mg |
| Calories from Fat | 15 | **Total Carbohydrate** | 14 g |
| **Total Fat** | 2.0 g | Dietary Fiber | 2 g |
| Saturated Fat | 0.3 g | Sugars | 0 g |
| Trans Fat | 0.0 g | Added Sugars | 3 g |
| **Cholesterol** | 0 mg | **Protein** | 3 g |
| **Sodium** | 5 mg | **Phosphorus** | 90 mg |

# Old-Fashioned Rolled Oats

SERVES 4 ■ SERVING SIZE 1/2 cup
PREP TIME 5 minutes ■ COOK TIME 10 minutes

1 cup old-fashioned rolled oats
2 cups water

1 Add the oats and water to a saucepan over high heat.

2 Bring to a boil, stirring constantly. Reduce heat to low and simmer; continue stirring for about 5 minutes, or until oats have thickened.

3 Store in an airtight container in the refrigerator for up to 1 week, or put 1-cup portions in freezer bags and store frozen for up to 6 months.

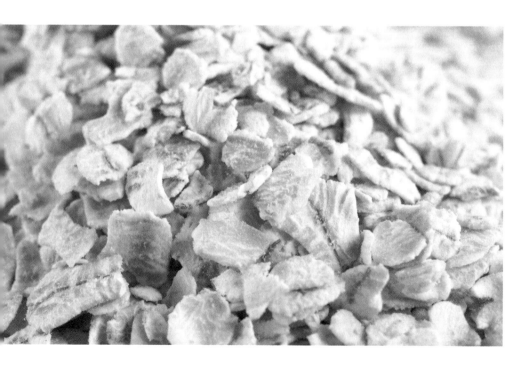

# Steel-Cut Oats

SERVES 4 ■ SERVING SIZE 1/2 cup
PREP TIME 5 minutes ■ COOK TIME 30 minutes

1 cup steel-cut oats
3 cups water

1 Add the oats and water to a saucepan over high heat.

2 Bring to a boil, stirring constantly. Reduce heat to low and simmer, uncovered, for about 30 minutes, stirring occasionally. The oats should be thick and creamy.

3 Store in an airtight container in the refrigerator for up to 1 week, or put 1-cup portions in freezer bags and store frozen for up to 6 months.

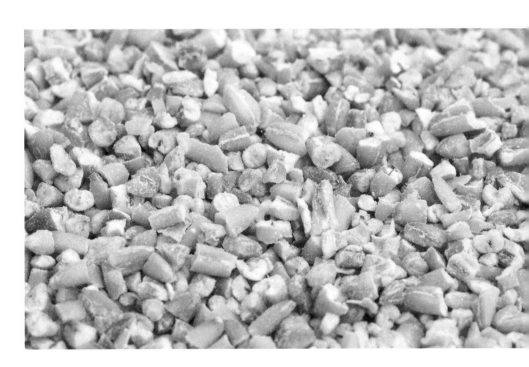

# Quick-Cooking Oats

SERVES 4 ■ SERVING SIZE 1/2 cup
PREP TIME 5 minutes ■ COOK TIME less than 5 minutes

1 cup quick-cooking oats

2 cups water

1 Add the oats and water to a saucepan on a stovetop over high heat.

2 Bring to a boil, stirring constantly, for about 1–2 minutes, or until oats have thickened.

3 Store in an airtight container in the refrigerator for up to 1 week, or put 1-cup portions in freezer bags and store frozen for up to 6 months.

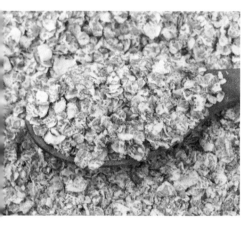

## WAYS TO USE COOKED OATMEAL

- Fruit-and-nut oatmeal: Stir in 1/4 cup berries and 1 Tablespoon toasted nuts to 1/2 cup cooked oatmeal (if you need it, sweeten with 1 teaspoon of honey or granulated sugar substitute such as Stevia)
- Banana bread oatmeal: Stir in 1/2 of a small mashed, ripe banana and 1 Tablespoon toasted walnuts to 1/2 cup cooked oatmeal.
- Oatmeal pudding: Use the recipe for Brown Rice Pudding on page 60 and substitute the cooked oatmeal for the cooked brown rice. Follow the rest of the instructions.
- Apple pie oatmeal: Top 1/2 cup cooked oatmeal with 1/4 cup chunky applesauce; 1 Tablespoon toasted, chopped walnuts; and a dusting of cinnamon.
- Fruit, oatmeal, and yogurt parfait: Layer 1/2 cup cooked oats with 1/3 cup low-fat blueberry yogurt, 1/4 cup fresh blueberries, and 2 Tablespoons reduced-sugar granola.

# Veggie and Oatmeal Stir-Fry

SERVES 2 ■ SERVING SIZE 3/4 cup
PREP TIME 15 minutes ■ COOK TIME 15 minutes

1 Tablespoon olive oil

1 cup sliced button mushrooms

2 cups baby spinach

1/2 cup frozen peas

1 clove garlic, minced or grated

2 teaspoons lower-sodium soy sauce

1/4 teaspoon ground black pepper

1 cup cooked Old-Fashioned Rolled Oatmeal (see recipe on page 62), set aside

**Optional ingredients:**

1/4 teaspoon crushed red pepper flakes

1 teaspoon Asian-style hot sauce, such as Sriracha

1 Add olive oil to a nonstick skillet over medium-high heat. Add mushrooms and sauté for 5–7 minutes until mushrooms are soft and most of the liquid in the pan has evaporated.

2 Add the spinach and sauté for 3–4 minutes or until the spinach is wilted. Turn the heat down to medium-low.

3 Add the peas, garlic, soy sauce, ground black pepper, and (if using) 1/4 teaspoon crushed red pepper flakes and 1 teaspoon Asian-style hot sauce. Sauté for 3–4 minutes and then stir in the cooked oatmeal and sauté to heat through, about 2–3 minutes.

## CHEF TIP

Enhance this dish even more by adding your leftover cooked protein such as cooked chicken, shrimp, or steak. Because you're using oatmeal, this dish is much higher in fiber than a stir-fry using white rice and it is a unique way to use up oatmeal.

**Choices/Exchanges**
1 Starch, 1 Nonstarchy Vegetable, 2 Fat

**Basic Nutritional Values**

| | |
|---|---|
| **Calories** | 190 |
| Calories from Fat | 80 |
| **Total Fat** | 9.0 g |
| Saturated Fat | 1.4 g |
| Trans Fat | 0.0 g |
| **Cholesterol** | 0 mg |
| **Sodium** | 230 mg |
| **Potassium** | 550 mg |
| **Total Carbohydrate** | 22 g |
| Dietary Fiber | 5 g |
| Sugars | 3 g |
| Added Sugars | 0 g |
| **Protein** | 7 g |
| **Phosphorus** | 165 mg |

# Basic Quinoa

SERVES 4 ▪ SERVING SIZE 1/2 cup
PREP TIME 5 minutes ▪ COOK TIME 25 minutes

Even though it is not technically a grain, quinoa is widely considered a great whole-grain option. This superfood is actually a complete protein and is high in fiber. You can use it in place of rice, oatmeal, barley, or couscous in any dish. It eats well both savory and sweet, and is simple to cook. Here is a basic recipe for cooking quinoa of any color, with some great ideas on how to use it.

1 cup quinoa
1 1/2 cups water

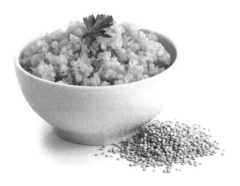

1 Add the dry quinoa to a mesh colander and rinse under cold running water.

2 Combine the rinsed quinoa and 1 1/2 cups water in a saucepan over high heat and bring to a boil.

3 Reduce to a simmer and cover. Cook the quinoa for 12–15 minutes until all the liquid is absorbed.

4 Turn off the heat and leave the lid on for 10 minutes to steam. Fluff the quinoa with a fork.

5 Store in an airtight container in the refrigerator for up to 1 week, or put 1-cup portions in freezer bags and store frozen for up to 6 months.

## WAYS TO USE

- Use as a starch side dish for any meat and vegetable.
- Replace rice, couscous, oatmeal, or barley in any dish (see options for rice on page 59, oatmeal on page 64, and barley on page 69).

**Choices/Exchanges**
1 1/2 Starch

**Basic Nutritional Values**

| | | | |
|---|---|---|---|
| **Calories** | 110 | **Potassium** | 210 mg |
| Calories from Fat | 15 | **Total Carbohydrate** | 20 g |
| **Total Fat** | 2.0 g | Dietary Fiber | 2.5 g |
| Saturated Fat | 0.2 g | Sugars | 1 g |
| Trans Fat | 0.0 g | Added Sugars | 0 g |
| **Cholesterol** | 0 mg | **Protein** | 4 g |
| **Sodium** | 5 mg | **Phosphorus** | 140 mg |

# Greek Quinoa Salad

SERVES 6 ■ SERVING SIZE 1/2 cup
PREP TIME 15 minutes ■ COOK TIME N/A

3 Tablespoons red wine vinegar

2 Tablespoons olive oil

1/2 teaspoon Dijon mustard

1/2 teaspoon dried dill

1/4 teaspoon salt

1/4 teaspoon ground black pepper

1 cup cucumber, medium dice

1 cup cherry or grape tomatoes, cut in half

1 cup bell pepper (any color), medium dice

1/4 cup crumbled feta cheese

1 cup cooked and cooled quinoa (see Basic Quinoa on page 66), set aside

1  In a medium bowl, whisk the red wine vinegar, olive oil, Dijon mustard, dried dill, salt, and pepper.

2  Add the cucumbers, tomatoes, bell pepper, and feta cheese. Gently stir the vegetables and cheese in the dressing to coat.

3  Add in the quinoa and gently stir to combine.

4  Store in an airtight container in the refrigerator for up to 1 week.

## CHEF TIP

You can use any vegetables you like in this dish. You can also change up the cheese. Try shredded Parmesan or crumbled blue cheese for a unique flavor. Strong-tasting cheeses are great in healthy cooking because you do not need to use a lot to get a big flavor impact on your dish.

**Choices/Exchanges**
1/2 Starch, 1 Nonstarchy Vegetable, 1 Fat

**Basic Nutritional Values**

| | |
|---|---|
| **Calories** | 110 |
| Calories from Fat | 50 |
| **Total Fat** | 6.0 g |
| Saturated Fat | 1.3 g |
| Trans Fat | 0.0 g |
| **Cholesterol** | 6 mg |
| **Sodium** | 160 mg |
| **Potassium** | 210 mg |
| **Total Carbohydrate** | 10 g |
| Dietary Fiber | 2 g |
| Sugars | 3 g |
| Added Sugars | 0 g |
| **Protein** | 3 g |
| **Phosphorus** | 80 mg |

# Basic Barley

SERVES 6 ▪ SERVING SIZE 1/2 cup
PREP TIME 5 minutes ▪ COOK TIME 55 minutes

Barley is an excellent whole grain that has a nutty, chewy texture. You can use it in place of any grain, including rice, quinoa, oatmeal, and pasta. Hulled barley is considered the whole-grain barley, and will have more nutrients and fiber and a better texture. Pearl barley is also delicious, but is not the whole grain. Like all grains, barley works well both savory and sweet, although it is traditionally used in more savory dishes.

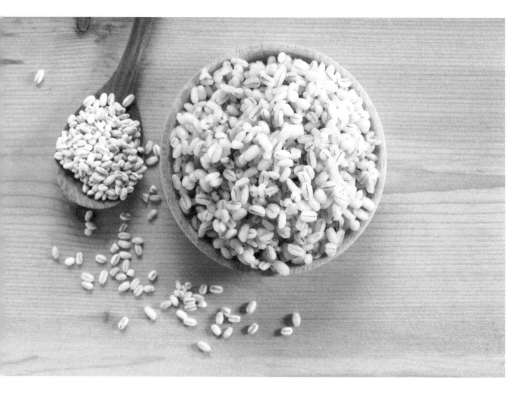

1 cup hulled barley

3 cups water

1 Combine the barley and water in a saucepan over high heat and bring to a boil.

2 Reduce to a simmer and cover. Cook the barley for 45 minutes.

3 Turn off the heat and leave the lid on for 10 minutes to steam. If there is water still in the pan, drain the barley.

4 Fluff with a fork.

5 Store in an airtight container in the refrigerator for up to 1 week, or put 1-cup portions in freezer bags and store frozen for up to 6 months.

## WAYS TO USE

- Use as a starch side dish for any meat and vegetable.
- Replace rice, couscous, oatmeal, or quinoa in any dish (see options for rice on page 59, oatmeal on page 64, and quinoa on page 66).

## CHEF TIP

Adding cooked barley to a dish like soup saves time and does not end up soaking up all of the cooking liquid that it would normally use if you cooked the barley in the soup. Plus, if you have the barley precooked and stored in the refrigerator and freezer, you will save about 1 hour of work during the week when you are looking for a quick meal!

**Choices/Exchanges**
1 1/2 Starch

**Basic Nutritional Values**

| | |
|---|---|
| **Calories** | 100 |
| Calories from Fat | 5 |
| **Total Fat** | <0.5 g |
| Saturated Fat | <0.1 g |
| Trans Fat | 0.0 g |
| **Cholesterol** | 0 mg |
| **Sodium** | 160 mg |
| **Potassium** | 80 mg |
| **Total Carbohydrate** | 24 g |
| Dietary Fiber | 3 g |
| Sugars | 0 g |
| Added Sugars | 0 g |
| **Protein** | 2 g |
| **Phosphorus** | 45 mg |

# Barley-Stuffed Peppers

SERVES 4 ■ SERVING SIZE 1/2 pepper with filling
PREP TIME 15 minutes ■ COOK TIME 30 minutes

Nonstick cooking spray

2 bell peppers, any color (recommend red bell pepper)

1 cup cooked barley (see Basic Barley on page 68), set aside

1 small onion, peeled and small dice (about 1 cup of diced onion)

2 (3-ounce) links precooked chicken sausage (any flavor), small diced (such as Al Fresco Sweet Italian Chicken Sausage)

1/4 cup grated Parmesan cheese

1/4 teaspoon salt

1/4 teaspoon ground black pepper

1 Preheat oven to 350°F. Coat a sheet pan with nonstick cooking spray. Set aside.

2 Cut the bell peppers in half lengthwise (vertically) and remove and discard the white ribs and seeds. Lay the peppers cut-side-up on the prepared sheet pan. Set aside.

3 In a bowl, mix together the cooked barley, onion, chicken sausage, Parmesan cheese, salt, and pepper.

**CHEF TIP**

Like it spicier? Use Poblano peppers instead of bell peppers and spicy chicken sausage for this recipe.

**Choices/Exchanges**
1 Starch, 1 Nonstarchy Vegetable, 1 Lean Protein

**Basic Nutritional Values**

| | |
|---|---|
| **Calories** | 160 |
| Calories from Fat | 45 |
| **Total Fat** | 5.0 g |
| Saturated Fat | 1.6 g |
| Trans Fat | 0.0 g |
| **Cholesterol** | 30 mg |
| **Sodium** | 460 mg |
| **Potassium** | 360 mg |
| **Total Carbohydrate** | 19 g |
| Dietary Fiber | 5 g |
| Sugars | 5 g |
| Added Sugars | 1 g |
| **Protein** | 11 g |
| **Phosphorus** | 175 mg |

4   Evenly distribute the barley filling into each pepper half.

5   Bake for 30 minutes in the pre-heated oven.

6   Remove from oven and serve, or store in an airtight container in the refrigerator for up to 1 week.

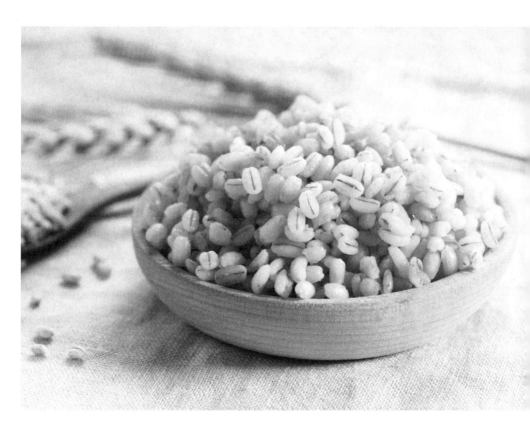

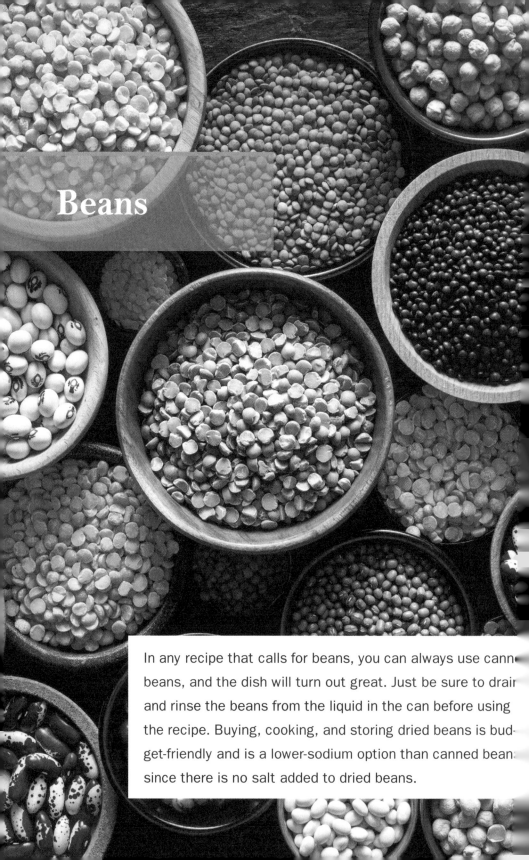

# Beans

In any recipe that calls for beans, you can always use canned beans, and the dish will turn out great. Just be sure to drain and rinse the beans from the liquid in the can before using the recipe. Buying, cooking, and storing dried beans is budget-friendly and is a lower-sodium option than canned beans since there is no salt added to dried beans.

# How to Cook Dried Beans

**SERVES** 10 ■ **SERVING SIZE** 1/2 cup cooked beans
**PREP TIME** 1 hour ■ **COOK TIME** 30–60 minutes,
depending on the bean size and type

This is a method for cooking dried beans that is a "quick" soaking method, rather than soaking beans overnight. You can always soak the beans in cold water and store in the refrigerator overnight, and skip the first step in this recipe.

12 cups water, divided

1 pound dried beans, such as
    pinto beans

1 Add 6 cups water to a stock pot over high heat and bring to a boil. Add the dried beans and boil rapidly for 2 minutes.

2 Remove the pot from the heat and cover. Let sit for 1 hour.

3 Drain and rinse the beans. Return them to the stock pot.

*(continued on next page)*

# How to Cook Dried Beans

*(continued)*

## HOW TO USE

- These beans can be used in any recipe calling for cooked or canned beans. One 15-ounce can of drained canned beans equals 1 1/2 cups of drained cooked dried beans.
- Replace meat in a taco, burrito, or quesadilla with beans for a great meatless option.
- Serve chilled in a salad.
- Layer with cooked brown rice, salsa, lettuce, cheese, and guacamole for a meatless burrito bowl.
- Add to soups and stews for added protein and fiber.
- Mash them with a little vegetable broth, garlic, and herbs and make a bean dip for fresh cut veggies or whole-grain pitas.

4 Add 6 fresh cups water to the beans in the stock pot and bring to a boil. Reduce to a simmer for up to 1 hour, or until the beans are soft but not split. This timing will vary based on the size and type of bean. Start checking the beans for doneness around 20 minutes.

5 Store in an airtight container in the refrigerator for up to 1 week, or put 1-cup portions in freezer bags and store frozen for up to 6 months.

**Choices/Exchanges**
1 1/2 Starch

**Basic Nutritional Values**

| | |
|---|---|
| **Calories** | 130 |
| Calories from Fat | 5 |
| **Total Fat** | <1.0 g |
| Saturated Fat | <0.1 g |
| Trans Fat | 0.0 g |
| **Cholesterol** | 0 mg |
| **Sodium** | 200 mg |
| **Potassium** | 390 mg |
| **Total Carbohydrate** | 23 g |
| Dietary Fiber | 8 g |
| Sugars | 0 g |
| Added Sugars | 0 g |
| **Protein** | 8 g |
| **Phosphorus** | 130 mg |

# Herby Bean Dip

SERVES 10 ■ SERVING SIZE 2 Tablespoons
PREP TIME 5 minutes ■ COOK TIME 0 minutes

1 1/2 cups cooked beans (such as pinto, cannellini, or great northern beans), or 1 (15-ounce) can of beans, drained and rinsed

1/4 cup water or low-sodium vegetable broth

1 clove garlic, minced or grated

1/4 cup chopped fresh herbs (any combination of parsley, chives, basil, dill, or mint, see Chef Tip for this recipe)

1/4 teaspoon ground black pepper

1 Add all ingredients to a bowl and mash with a fork or potato masher to combine.

2 Serve with cut-up raw vegetables or whole-grain tortilla chips or crackers, or use as a sandwich or wrap filling.

## CHEF TIP

If you don't have access to fresh herbs, you can always use celery leaves or the green part of scallions (green onions) as a substitute. This is a great way to use these leftover parts so they don't go to waste.

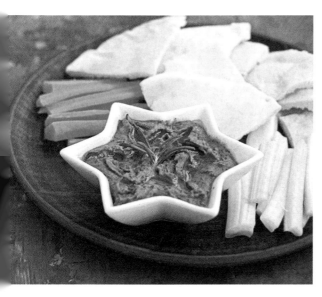

**Choices/Exchanges**
1/2 Starch

**Basic Nutritional Values**

| | |
|---|---|
| **Calories** | 35 |
| Calories from Fat | 0 |
| **Total Fat** | 0.0 g |
| Saturated Fat | 0.0 g |
| Trans Fat | 0.0 g |
| **Cholesterol** | 0 mg |
| **Sodium** | 0 mg |
| **Potassium** | 120 mg |
| **Total Carbohydrate** | 7 g |
| Dietary Fiber | 2 g |
| Sugars | 0 g |
| Added Sugars | 0 g |
| **Protein** | 2 g |
| **Phosphorus** | 40 mg |

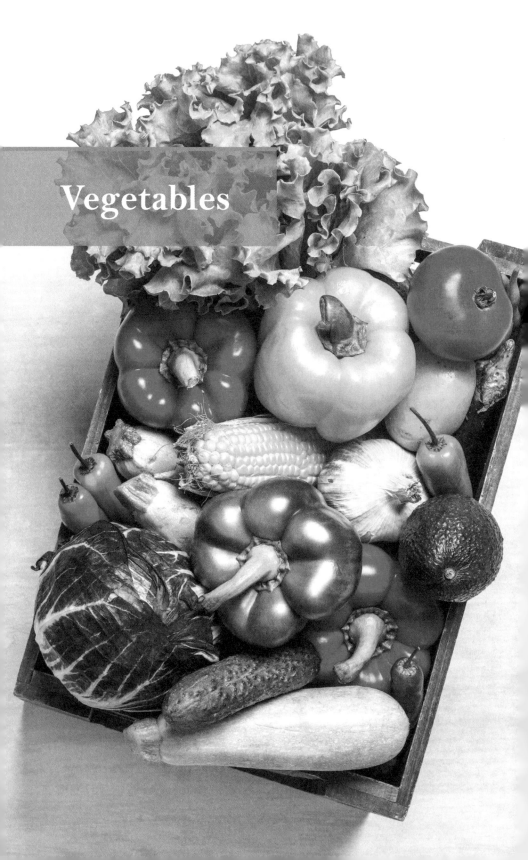

# Vegetables

Vegetables are a vital ingredient to any well-balanced meal. They can be prepared in a variety of ways—not just salads! Remember, try to fill half your plate with vegetables. You can incorporate vegetables into every meal by serving them on the side or incorporating them into the main dish.

Vegetables that taste great raw can be used for dipping in low-fat ranch dressing, bean dip, or hummus. They can be chopped up in a salad, stuffed into a wrap, layered on a sandwich, or just eaten as is. These vegetables include (but are not limited to):

- Cucumbers
- Bell peppers
- Carrots
- Celery
- Cauliflower
- Broccoli
- Cherry or grape tomatoes
- Snap peas

With the exception of cucumbers, all of these vegetables taste great cooked, too (especially roasted). Roasting vegetables is an excellent way to bring out their natural sweetness, and roasting makes vegetables easier to digest and more versatile to use in recipes. Once you have a batch of roasted vegetables, you can use them in countless way. Try the Roasted Vegetables recipe on the next page and all of its variations with your favorite veggies.

# Roasted Vegetables

SERVES 8 ■ SERVING SIZE 1/2 cup
PREP TIME 15 minutes ■ COOK TIME 45 minutes

Nonstick cooking spray

8 cups assorted vegetables, cut into equal inch-sized pieces (such as broccoli, cauliflower, bell pepper, onion, and mushrooms)

2 Tablespoons olive oil

1/4 teaspoon salt

1/2 teaspoon ground black pepper

1 Preheat the oven to 375°F. Spray a sheet pan with nonstick cooking spray, set aside.

2 In a bowl, mix together the vegetables, oil, salt, and pepper. Pour the mixture onto the sheet pan. Vegetables should be in a single layer. If the pan isn't big enough for all of the vegetables, use another sheet pan sprayed with nonstick cooking spray or cook in batches.

3 Bake for 40–45 minutes, stirring occasionally, until the vegetables are golden brown and tender.

4 Store in an airtight container in the refrigerator for up to 1 week, or put 1-cup portions in freezer bags and store frozen for up to 6 months.

## WAYS TO USE

- Eat as a side dish with grilled chicken or fish.
- Stir in to Scrambled Eggs (see page 54).
- Purée with chicken or vegetable broth to make a soup.
- Mix with canned or cooked dried beans (see "How to Cook Dried Beans" on page 73) or lentils.
- Serve chilled on a salad (see Roasted Vegetable Salad on page 78).
- Use as a filling for tacos, enchiladas, burritos, or quesadillas.
- Use as a topping for a roasted sweet potato (see Quick "Baked" Sweet Potato on page 83).

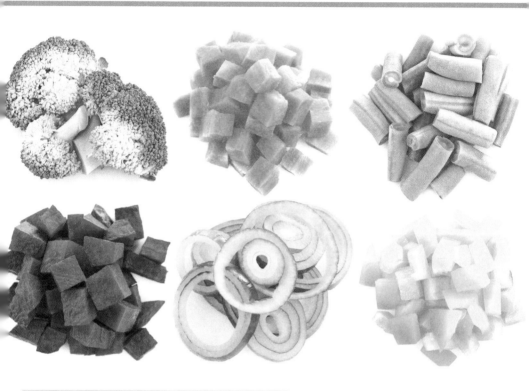

## VEGETABLES THAT ARE GREAT FOR ROASTING

- Asparagus
- Bell peppers
- Broccoli
- Brussels sprouts
- Cauliflower
- Celery
- Green beans
- Mushrooms
- Onions
- Tomatoes

**Choices/Exchanges**
1 Nonstarchy Vegetable, 1 Fat

**Basic Nutritional Values**

| | |
|---|---|
| **Calories** | 60 |
| Calories from Fat | 30 |
| **Total Fat** | 3.5 g |
| Saturated Fat | 0.5 g |
| Trans Fat | 0.0 g |
| **Cholesterol** | 0 mg |
| **Sodium** | 85 mg |
| **Potassium** | 250 mg |
| **Total Carbohydrate** | 6 g |
| Dietary Fiber | 2 g |
| Sugars | 3 g |
| Added Sugars | 0 g |
| **Protein** | 2 g |
| **Phosphorus** | 45 mg |

# Roasted Vegetable Salad

SERVES 1 ▪ SERVING SIZE 1 salad
PREP TIME 5 minutes ▪ COOK TIME 0 minutes

1/2 cup Roasted Vegetables (see page 78), chilled, set aside

1 cup baby lettuce greens

1 1/2 Tablespoons crumbled goat cheese

2 teaspoons roasted sunflower seeds

1 teaspoon fresh lemon juice

Pinch ground black pepper

1 Add all ingredients to a bowl and gently toss together.

2 Serve immediately.

## CHEF TIP

If you are packing this for your lunch, leave the lettuce separate from the rest of the ingredients until it's time to eat. You can toss all of the other ingredients together ahead of time and then serve on top of the lettuce.

**Choices/Exchanges**
2 Nonstarchy Vegetable, 2 Fat

**Basic Nutritional Values**

| | |
|---|---|
| **Calories** | 130 |
| Calories from Fat | 80 |
| **Total Fat** | 9.0 g |
| Saturated Fat | 2.4 g |
| Trans Fat | 0.0 g |
| **Cholesterol** | 10 mg |
| **Sodium** | 160 mg |
| **Potassium** | 390 mg |
| **Total Carbohydrate** | 9 g |
| Dietary Fiber | 4 g |
| Sugars | 4 g |
| Added Sugars | 0 g |
| **Protein** | 6 g |
| **Phosphorus** | 145 mg |

# Basic Spaghetti Squash

SERVES 4 ■ SERVING SIZE 1 cup
PREP TIME 10 minutes ■ COOK TIME 1 hour

Nonstick cooking spray

1 large spaghetti squash
(about 3-4 pounds)

## CHEF TIP

If you are having trouble cutting the raw spaghetti squash in half, try microwaving it first. Pierce the skin in several places with a fork, then microwave whole for about 4-5 minutes. This will soften the squash and make it easier to cut through.

1 Preheat oven to 375°F. Coat a sheet pan with nonstick cooking spray and set aside.

2 Cut the spaghetti squash in half lengthwise (vertically). Scoop out the seeds and discard, then place the squash halves cut side down on the sheet pan.

3 Bake for 45–60 minutes or until the squash is fork tender.

4 Remove from the oven and let cool. When the squash is cool enough to handle, rake a fork across the squash flesh to loosen the squash strands and remove from the skin. Discard the skin and put the squash "noodles" into a bowl.

5 Use in recipes calling for cooked spaghetti squash.

6 Store in an airtight container in the refrigerator for up to 1 week.

Choices/Exchanges
2 Nonstarchy Vegetable

Basic Nutritional Values

| Calories | 40 | | Potassium | 180 | mg |
|---|---|---|---|---|---|
| Calories from Fat | 0 | | Total Carbohydrate | 10 | g |
| Total Fat | 0.0 | g | Dietary Fiber | 2 | g |
| Saturated Fat | 0.1 | g | Sugars | 4 | g |
| Trans Fat | 0.0 | g | Added Sugars | 0 | g |
| Cholesterol | 0 | mg | Protein | 1 | g |
| Sodium | 30 | mg | Phosphorus | 20 | mg |

# Spaghetti Squash Cacio e Pepe

SERVES 4 ▪ SERVING SIZE 1 cup
PREP TIME 5 minutes ▪ COOK TIME 5 minutes

Cacio e Pepe is a simple pasta dish seasoned with garlic, Parmesan cheese, and black pepper. Here, we use spaghetti squash for a low-carb side dish. Add chicken and more vegetables for an entrée.

2 Tablespoons olive oil

3 cloves garlic, minced or grated

4 cups cooked spaghetti squash (about 1 whole squash)

1/4 cup grated Parmesan cheese

1/4 teaspoon salt

1/4 teaspoon ground black pepper

2 Tablespoons chopped fresh parsley

1 In a nonstick skillet, heat the olive oil over medium heat. Add the garlic and cook for 30 seconds. Add in the cooked spaghetti squash. Gently stir or toss to coat. Cook for 2–3 minutes in the olive oil and garlic.

2 Add the cheese, salt, and pepper. Toss or stir again to coat.

3 Garnish with chopped parsley. Serve immediately or store in an airtight container in the refrigerator for up to 1 week.

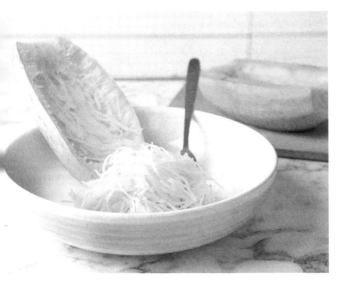

**Choices/Exchanges**
2 Nonstarchy Vegetable,
1 1/2 Fat

**Basic Nutritional Values**

| | |
|---|---|
| **Calories** | 120 |
| Calories from Fat | 70 |
| **Total Fat** | 8.0 g |
| Saturated Fat | 1.8 g |
| Trans Fat | 0.0 g |
| **Cholesterol** | 8 mg |
| **Sodium** | 240 mg |
| **Potassium** | 200 mg |
| **Total Carbohydrate** | 11 g |
| Dietary Fiber | 2 g |
| Sugars | 4 g |
| Added Sugars | 0 g |
| **Protein** | 3 g |
| **Phosphorus** | 55 mg |

# Quick "Baked" Sweet Potatoes

**SERVES** 4 ■ **SERVING SIZE** 1 medium sweet potato
**PREP TIME** 5 minutes ■ **COOK TIME** 20 minutes

4 medium sweet potatoes

1 Scrub and dry each sweet potato.

2 Pierce each sweet potato with a fork in a few spots.

3 Place the potatoes on a microwave-safe plate and microwave until fork tender, about 12–15 minutes.

4 Store in an airtight container in the refrigerator for up to 1 week or peel the sweet potato and store the flesh in a freezer bag or container and freeze up to 6 months.

## WAYS TO USE

- Cut open and stuff with a variety of ingredients such as Roasted Vegetables (see page 78), salsa, or chili (see Easy Turkey Chili on page 119).
- Use as a side dish with a protein and vegetable serving.
- Peel and cube and serve cold on a salad.
- Peel and cube and use as a base in a burrito bowl. Layer with taco meat, cheese, lettuce, salsa, and guacamole.
- Peel and cube and use in place of rice, oatmeal, barley, quinoa, or pasta in recipes.

**Choices/Exchanges**
1 1/2 Starch

**Basic Nutritional Values**

| | |
|---|---|
| **Calories** | 100 |
| Calories from Fat | 0 |
| **Total Fat** | 0.0 g |
| Saturated Fat | 0.0 g |
| Trans Fat | 0.0 g |
| **Cholesterol** | 0 mg |
| **Sodium** | 40 mg |
| **Potassium** | 200 mg |
| **Total Carbohydrate** | 23 g |
| Dietary Fiber | 4 g |
| Sugars | 7 g |
| Added Sugars | 0 g |
| **Protein** | 2 g |
| **Phosphorus** | 60 mg |

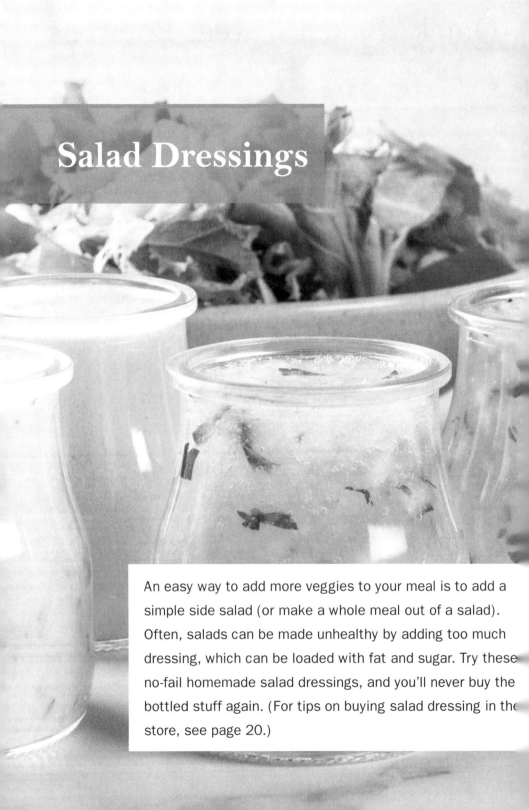

# Salad Dressings

An easy way to add more veggies to your meal is to add a simple side salad (or make a whole meal out of a salad). Often, salads can be made unhealthy by adding too much dressing, which can be loaded with fat and sugar. Try these no-fail homemade salad dressings, and you'll never buy the bottled stuff again. (For tips on buying salad dressing in the store, see page 20.)

# Easy Vinaigrette

1/4 cup red wine vinegar

1/2 cup olive oil

1 clove garlic, minced or grated

1 teaspoon Dijon mustard

1 Tablespoon honey or granulated sugar substitute such as Stevia

1/4 teaspoon ground black pepper

*Optional ingredients:*

1 Tablespoon chopped fresh oregano or 1/2 teaspoon dried oregano

1 Add all ingredients to a dressing shaker or Mason jar.

2 Shake well until combined.

3 Store in the refrigerator for up to 2 weeks. The olive oil and vinegar will separate over time—shake well before each use to mix everything together again.

## CHEF TIP

You can use any vinegar or citrus juice for this recipe and change up the flavor by adding different fresh herbs. Try the following combinations:

■ Balsamic vinegar and 1 Tablespoon chopped fresh basil or 1/2 teaspoon dried basil

■ Fresh lemon juice and 1 Tablespoon chopped fresh parsley or 1/2 teaspoon dried parsley

■ White wine vinegar and 1 Tablespoon chopped fresh chives or scallion greens

■ Fresh lime juice and 1 Tablespoon chopped fresh cilantro

**Choices/Exchanges**
3 Fat

**Basic Nutritional Values**

| | |
|---|---|
| **Calories** | 130 |
| Calories from Fat | 130 |
| **Total Fat** | 14.0 g |
| Saturated Fat | 1.9 g |
| Trans Fat | 0.0 g |
| **Cholesterol** | 0 mg |
| **Sodium** | 15 mg |
| **Potassium** | 10 mg |
| **Total Carbohydrate** | 2 g |
| Dietary Fiber | 0 g |
| Sugars | 2 g |
| Added Sugars | 2 g |
| **Protein** | 0 g |
| **Phosphorus** | 0 mg |

# Creamiest Ranch

SERVES 12 ■ SERVING SIZE 2 Tablespoons
PREP TIME 5 minutes ■ COOK TIME 0 minutes

1 cup low-fat buttermilk

1/2 cup fat-free, plain Greek yogurt

2 Tablespoons light mayonnaise

1 Tablespoon Dijon mustard

1 teaspoon onion powder

1 teaspoon dried dill

1 teaspoon dried parsley

1/4 teaspoon garlic powder

1/4 teaspoon ground black pepper

1 Whisk all ingredients in a bowl.

2 Transfer to a dressing shaker or Mason jar.

3 Store in the refrigerator for up to 1 week.

**Choices/Exchanges**
None

**Basic Nutritional Values**

| | |
|---|---|
| **Calories** | 20 |
| Calories from Fat | 10 |
| **Total Fat** | 1.0 g |
| Saturated Fat | 0.2 g |
| Trans Fat | 0.0 g |
| **Cholesterol** | 0 mg |
| **Sodium** | 70 mg |
| **Potassium** | 55 mg |
| **Total Carbohydrate** | 2 g |
| Dietary Fiber | 0 g |
| Sugars | 1 g |
| Added Sugars | 0 g |
| **Protein** | 2 g |
| **Phosphorus** | 35 mg |

# Green Goddess Dressing

SERVES 14 ■ SERVING SIZE 2 Tablespoons
PREP TIME 5 minutes ■ COOK TIME 0 minutes

4 scallions (green onions), white and green part, trimmed of root

1 cup parsley leaves

1 Creamiest Ranch recipe (see page 86), set aside

1 Tablespoon white wine vinegar

1. To make in a food processor or blender: add all ingredients to the pitcher or bowl and blend or process on high until the greens are puréed and the dressing is well-blended.

2. To make by hand: Mince the scallions and parsley until finely chopped. Add to a bowl with the Creamiest Ranch dressing and the white wine vinegar, and whisk to combine.

3. Transfer to a dressing shaker or Mason jar. Store in the refrigerator for up to 1 week.

**CHEF TIP**

Chef Tip: This dressing also makes a great dip for cut-up veggies or whole-grain pita chips.

**Choices/Exchanges**
None

**Basic Nutritional Values**

| | |
|---|---|
| **Calories** | 20 |
| Calories from Fat | 5 |
| **Total Fat** | 0.5 g |
| Saturated Fat | 0.2 g |
| Trans Fat | 0.0 g |
| **Cholesterol** | 0 mg |
| **Sodium** | 65 mg |
| **Potassium** | 80 mg |
| **Total Carbohydrate** | 2 g |
| Dietary Fiber | 0 g |
| Sugars | 1 g |
| Added Sugars | 0 g |
| **Protein** | 2 g |
| **Phosphorus** | 35 mg |

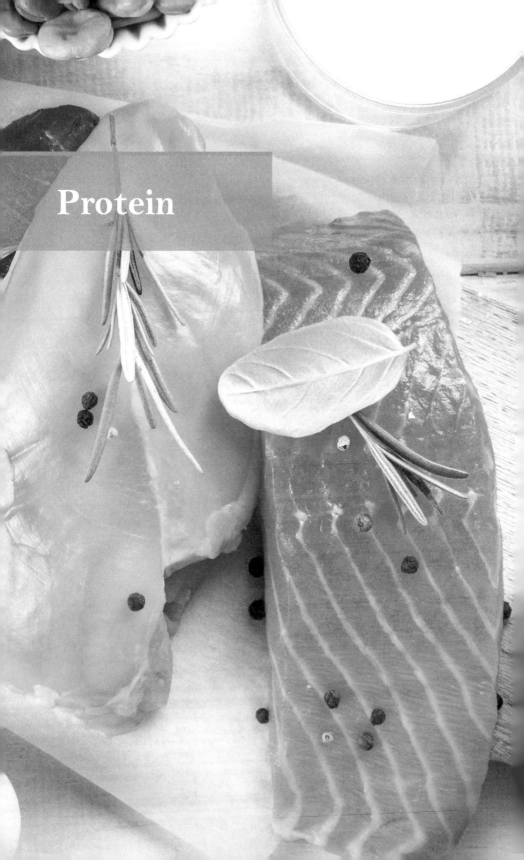

# Protein

# Chicken

Chicken is one of the most budget-friendly and diabetes-friendly meats available. Cooking a chicken ahead of time and using it throughout the week is quick and can help save you money. There are many recipes using cooked chicken throughout this book. While you can certainly use chicken already cooked from the grocery store, such as a rotisserie chicken, the sodium content is usually very high. These two methods for cooking a whole chicken will yield plenty of meat and broth with no added sodium at about half the price you'll pay for premade chicken. If a whole chicken seems like too much, we also show you how to cook juicy, flavorful chicken breasts.

# Whole Roasted Chicken

SERVES 12 ■ SERVING SIZE 1/2 cup shredded meat
PREP TIME 5 minutes ■ COOK TIME 65 minutes

Nonstick cooking spray
1 (5-pound) whole chicken

1 Preheat oven to 450°F. Coat a 9 × 13 baking dish with nonstick cooking spray.

2 Remove the giblet and neck from chicken cavity (discard, or save for making chicken broth). Pat the skin dry with a paper towel.

3 Place chicken breast-side-up into the pan and lightly spray the skin with nonstick cooking spray.

4 Bake in oven for 20 minutes. After 20 minutes, reduce heat to 350°F and bake chicken an additional 45 minutes or until the internal temperature of the thigh meat is 165°F.

5 Remove the chicken from the pan and let it rest on a cutting board, covered with foil for 20 minutes.

6 Once the chicken has rested, remove and discard the skin and carve or pull all of the meat from the bones.

7 Save the carcass (bones) and use it for making chicken broth (see page 94 for instructions).

8 Store the meat in an airtight container in the refrigerator for up to 1 week, or pack in freezer bags or containers and store in the freezer up to 3 months.

## CHEF TIP

To take the internal temperature of chicken, use an instant-read thermometer inserted into the thickest part of the thigh, but do not let the thermometer touch bone. The breast meat cooks faster than the thigh meat, and you'll want to ensure the whole chicken is cooked to 165°F (safe temperature of doneness for chicken) before serving. Consuming raw or undercooked meats, poultry, seafood, shellfish, or eggs may increase your risk of foodborne illness.

**Choices/Exchanges**
2 Lean Protein

**Basic Nutritional Values**

| | |
|---|---|
| **Calories** | 115 |
| Calories from Fat | 45 |
| **Total Fat** | 5.0 g |
| Saturated Fat | 1.2 g |
| Trans Fat | 0.0 g |
| **Cholesterol** | 50 mg |
| **Sodium** | 50 mg |
| **Potassium** | 160 mg |
| **Total Carbohydrate** | 0 g |
| Dietary Fiber | 0 g |
| Sugars | 0 g |
| Added Sugars | 0 g |
| **Protein** | 18 g |
| **Phosphorus** | 135 mg |

# Simmered Chicken and Broth

SERVES 12 ■ SERVING SIZE 1/2 cup shredded meat
PREP TIME 5 minutes ■ COOK TIME 90 minutes

1 (5-pound) whole chicken
1 onion, peeled and chopped
1 large carrot, peeled and chopped
2 ribs of celery, chopped
Water

**Choices/Exchanges**
2 Lean Protein

**Basic Nutritional Values**

| | |
|---|---|
| **Calories** | 115 |
| Calories from Fat | 45 |
| **Total Fat** | 5.0 g |
| Saturated Fat | 1.2 g |
| Trans Fat | 0.0 g |
| **Cholesterol** | 50 mg |
| **Sodium** | 50 mg |
| **Potassium** | 160 mg |
| **Total Carbohydrate** | 0 g |
| Dietary Fiber | 0 g |
| Sugars | 0 g |
| Added Sugars | 0 g |
| **Protein** | 18 g |
| **Phosphorus** | 135 mg |

1 Remove the giblet and neck from chicken cavity (discard, or add to the pot to flavor the broth). Place the chicken in a large stock pot and add the onions, carrots, and celery. Add enough cold water to the pot so that the water is 2 inches above the chicken and vegetables.

2 Bring to a boil and then reduce to a gentle simmer for 90 minutes.

3 Remove the chicken from the broth and set aside to cool slightly on a cutting board or in a large bowl.

4 Strain the broth using a mesh colander into a bowl. Store the broth in an airtight container in the refrigerator for up to 1 week or pack in freezer bags or containers and store in the freezer up to 6 months (leave at least 1/2-inch of space at the top of a container—the broth will expand as it freezes).

5 Once the chicken has rested, remove and discard the skin and carve or pull all of the meat from the bones. Store the chicken meat in an airtight container in the refrigerator for up to 1 week or pack in freezer bags or containers and store in the freezer up to 3 months. Discard the carcass, or save for making more chicken broth (see instructions on page 94).

# Simple Chicken Breast

SERVES 4 ■ SERVING SIZE 3 ounces
PREP TIME 5 minutes ■ COOK TIME 20–25 minutes

Nonstick cooking spray

1 pound boneless, skinless chicken breasts

1/2 teaspoon salt

1/2 teaspoon ground black pepper

1 Preheat oven to 400°F. Coat a baking sheet with nonstick cooking spray.

2 Place the chicken breasts on the prepared baking sheets and lightly coat the tops of the chicken with two sprays of nonstick cooking spray. Season with salt and pepper.

3 Bake for 20–25 minutes or until the internal temperature reaches 165°F.

4 Remove from the oven and place the chicken breasts on a cutting board. Let them rest for 10 minutes before cutting, or cool and store whole in the refrigerator for up to 1 week or in the freezer for up to 3 months. Do not slice until ready to serve to retain moisture.

**CHEF TIP**
You can change up the flavor of this chicken with a squeeze of fresh lemon or lime juice, garlic or onion powder, dried herbs, or no-salt-added seasoning.

**Choices/Exchanges**
3 Lean Protein

**Basic Nutritional Values**

| | |
|---|---|
| **Calories** | 120 |
| Calories from Fat | 45 |
| **Total Fat** | 3.0 g |
| Saturated Fat | 0.5 g |
| Trans Fat | 0.0 g |
| **Cholesterol** | 75 mg |
| **Sodium** | 350 mg |
| **Potassium** | 240 mg |
| **Total Carbohydrate** | 0 g |
| Dietary Fiber | 0 g |
| Sugars | 0 g |
| Added Sugars | 0 g |
| **Protein** | 24 g |
| **Phosphorus** | 210 mg |

# How to Make Chicken Broth

Don't throw away the carcass! Whether you cooked a whole chicken at home, or purchased a rotisserie chicken from the store, you can use the leftover bones to make a simple, salt-free chicken broth. Simply throw all of the bones and scraps into a large pot with some roughly chopped vegetables or vegetable scraps and enough water to cover everything by 1–2 inches. Bring everything to a boil, then reduce to a simmer. Cover the pot and simmer for at least 30 minutes (or up to several hours).

Let the broth cool, then strain out the solids with a mesh colander. Store in an airtight container (divide into multiple containers if needed) in the refrigerator for up to 1 week, or in the freezer for up to 6 months. If you are freezing the broth, leave at least a half-inch of space in the container—the broth will expand as it freezes.

Traditional broth is made with carrots, onion, and celery, but you could also add garlic, peppers, leeks, dried or fresh herbs, and spices like black peppercorns. For even more flavor, roast the vegetables for your broth before adding to the pot (if you are roasting a chicken at home, you can roast vegetables for the broth alongside the chicken).

Don't add salt to your homemade broth! When you make soup or other dishes with the broth, you will have more control over how much salt ends up in the finished dish.

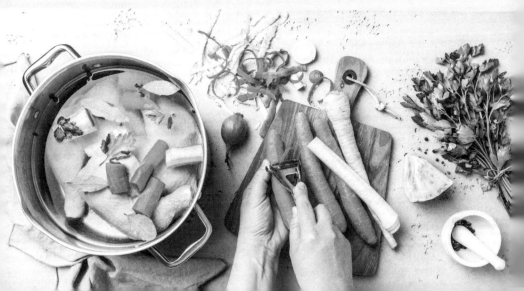

# Open-Face Chicken Salad Sandwich

SERVES 4 ■ SERVING SIZE 1 toast with 1/2 cup chicken salad
PREP TIME 10 minutes ■ COOK TIME 0 minutes

2 cups cooked, shredded chicken

1/4 cup light mayonnaise

1/4 cup fat-free, plain Greek yogurt

2 Tablespoons minced onion

1/4 teaspoon salt

1/4 teaspoon ground black pepper

1 teaspoon dried dill

4 pieces whole-wheat bread, toasted

1/4 cup toasted slivered almonds

1 In a bowl, mix together the chicken, light mayonnaise, Greek yogurt, minced onion, salt, pepper, and dried dill.

2 Top one piece of toast with 1/2 cup chicken salad mix. Top with 1 Tablespoon toasted slivered almonds.

3 Repeat for remaining three pieces of toast. Or, store the chicken salad separate from the nuts in an airtight container in the refrigerator for up to 1 week, and assemble the open-faced sandwiches as needed.

**Choices/Exchanges**
1 Starch, 1/2 Carbohydrate, 3 Lean Protein, 1 1/2 Fat

**Basic Nutritional Values**

| | |
|---|---|
| **Calories** | 320 |
| Calories from Fat | 120 |
| **Total Fat** | 13.0 g |
| Saturated Fat | 2.0 g |
| Trans Fat | 0.0 g |
| **Cholesterol** | 65 mg |
| **Sodium** | 500 mg |
| **Potassium** | 330 mg |
| **Total Carbohydrate** | 23 g |
| Dietary Fiber | 3 g |
| Sugars | 5 g |
| Added Sugars | 3 g |
| **Protein** | 28 g |
| **Phosphorus** | 285 mg |

**CHEF TIP**
Swap out the toast for a lettuce leaf to make a low-carb, chicken-salad lettuce wrap.

# Chicken and Spaghetti Squash Parmesan

SERVES 6 ■ SERVING SIZE 1 cup
PREP TIME 10 minutes ■ COOK TIME 25 minutes

4 cups cooked spaghetti squash (see Basic Spaghetti Squash recipe, page 81), set aside

2 cups cooked, shredded chicken

Nonstick cooking spray

2 cups no-sugar-added jarred pasta sauce (such as Prego No-Sugar-Added Traditional Italian Sauce)

1/4 cup grated Parmesan cheese

1/4 cup low-moisture, part-skim mozzarella cheese

1 Preheat oven to 375°F. Coat a 9 × 13 baking dish with nonstick cooking spray, set aside.

2 Layer the spaghetti squash on the bottom of the baking dish. Evenly place the chicken over the squash and then cover with the pasta sauce.

3 Sprinkle the Parmesan and mozzarella cheeses over the sauce.

4 Bake for 25 minutes, or until the cheese on top is melted and slightly browned. Let cool slightly before serving.

5 Store cooled leftovers in an airtight container in the refrigerator for up to 1 week.

**CHEF TIP**
Make this dish a little spicier by adding 1 teaspoon crushed red pepper flakes to the sauce before pouring on top of the chicken.

**Choices/Exchanges**
1/2 Starch, 1 Nonstarchy Vegetable, 2 Lean Protein, 1/2 Fat

**Basic Nutritional Values**

| | |
|---|---|
| **Calories** | 180 |
| Calories from Fat | 60 |
| **Total Fat** | 7.0 g |
| Saturated Fat | 2.1 g |
| Trans Fat | 0.0 g |
| **Cholesterol** | 45 mg |
| **Sodium** | 430 mg |
| **Potassium** | 510 mg |
| **Total Carbohydrate** | 13 g |
| Dietary Fiber | 3 g |
| Sugars | 7 g |
| Added Sugars | 0 g |
| **Protein** | 18 g |
| **Phosphorus** | 180 mg |

# Chicken Lettuce Wraps

SERVES 4 ■ SERVING SIZE 1 lettuce wrap
PREP TIME 10 minutes ■ COOK TIME 0 minutes

1 1/2 cups cooked, shredded chicken

3 scallions (green onions), green and white parts, chopped

2 Tablespoons chopped roasted peanuts

2 Tablespoons lower-sodium soy sauce

1/2 teaspoon ground black pepper

1 8-ounce can sliced water chestnuts, drained

4 large butter lettuce leaves

1 In a bowl, mix together the chicken, scallions, peanuts, soy sauce, black pepper, and water chestnuts.

2 Fill each lettuce leaf with 1/2 cup of chicken mixture.

3 To prepare and store for later, store the chicken mixture separate from the lettuce leaves in an airtight container in the refrigerator for up to 1 week. Assemble as needed.

**Choices/Exchanges**
1 Nonstarchy Vegetable, 2 Lean Protein, 1 Fat

**Basic Nutritional Values**

| | |
|---|---|
| **Calories** | 170 |
| Calories from Fat | 50 |
| **Total Fat** | 6.0 g |
| Saturated Fat | 1.4 g |
| Trans Fat | 0.0 g |
| **Cholesterol** | 45 mg |
| **Sodium** | 370 mg |
| **Potassium** | 530 mg |
| **Total Carbohydrate** | 8 g |
| Dietary Fiber | 2 g |
| Sugars | 2 g |
| Added Sugars | 0 g |
| **Protein** | 18 g |
| **Phosphorus** | 150 mg |

# Chicken and Veggie Stir-Fry

SERVES 4 ■ SERVING SIZE 1 1/2 cups
PREP TIME 10 minutes ■ COOK TIME 10 minutes

1 cup low-sodium chicken or vegetable broth

2 Tablespoons lower-sodium soy sauce

2 teaspoons cornstarch

1 clove garlic, minced or grated

1/2 teaspoon ground black pepper

1 Tablespoon olive oil

1 14-ounce bag frozen stir-fry vegetables

1 1/2 cups shredded, cooked chicken

1 Whisk the broth, soy sauce, cornstarch, garlic, and black pepper in a bowl until combined. Set aside.

2 Add olive oil to a nonstick skillet over high heat. Add the frozen vegetables and sauté for 5–7 minutes, stirring frequently.

3 Add the chicken and sauce to the pan and sauté another 5–7 minutes, until chicken is heated through and sauce is thickened.

**Choices/Exchanges**
2 Nonstarchy Vegetable, 2 Lean Protein, 1 Fat

**Basic Nutritional Values**

| | |
|---|---|
| **Calories** | 180 |
| Calories from Fat | 70 |
| **Total Fat** | 8.0 g |
| Saturated Fat | 1.6 g |
| Trans Fat | 0.0 g |
| **Cholesterol** | 45 mg |
| **Sodium** | 380 mg |
| **Potassium** | 530 mg |
| **Total Carbohydrate** | 9 g |
| Dietary Fiber | 2 g |
| Sugars | 3 g |
| Added Sugars | 0 g |
| **Protein** | 18 g |
| **Phosphorus** | 195 mg |

4 Serve over a whole grain like brown rice or quinoa, or over cauliflower rice for a low-carb dish.

5 Store cooled leftovers in an airtight container in the refrigerator for up to 1 week.

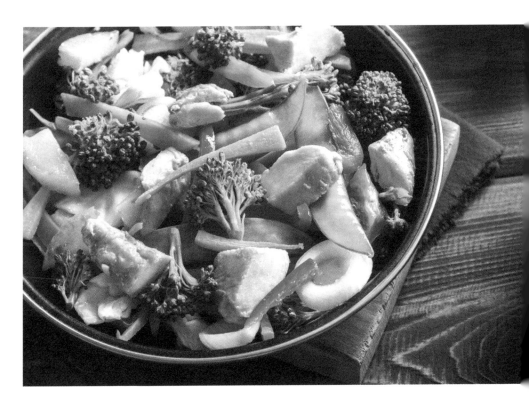

# Chicken and Spinach Pizza

**SERVES** 2 ■ **SERVING SIZE** 1 individual pizza
**PREP TIME** 10 minutes ■ **COOK TIME** 25 minutes

Nonstick cooking spray

2 teaspoons olive oil

2 cups baby spinach

2 cloves garlic, minced or grated

1/2 cup no-sugar-added pasta sauce

1/2 cup cooked, shredded chicken

1/4 teaspoon ground black pepper

1 whole-wheat pocket pita

3 Tablespoons low-moisture, part-skim mozzarella cheese, divided

1 Tablespoon grated Parmesan cheese, divided

1 Preheat oven to 375°F. Coat a sheet pan with nonstick cooking spray. Set aside.

2 Add olive oil to a nonstick sauté pan over medium-high heat. Add the spinach and garlic and sauté for 5 minutes or until spinach is wilted.

3 Add the pasta sauce and cook for 2 minutes.

4 Add the chicken and pepper. Stir to combine and remove from the heat.

5 Split the pita in half horizontally to end up with two circular pita halves. Lay the pitas on the prepared baking sheet cut-side-up. Divide the chicken mixture evenly between the two pitas.

6 Sprinkle 1 1/2 Tablespoons mozzarella cheese and 1 1/2 teaspoon Parmesan cheese evenly on top of each pita pizza.

7 Bake in the oven for 15 minutes or until cheese is golden brown.

8 Remove from oven and cut each pizza into quarters. Serve hot.

**Choices/Exchanges**
1 Starch, 1 Nonstarchy Vegetable, 2 Lean Protein, 1 1/2 Fat

**Basic Nutritional Values**

| | |
|---|---|
| **Calories** | 270 |
| Calories from Fat | 100 |
| **Total Fat** | 11.0 g |
| Saturated Fat | 3.1 g |
| Trans Fat | 0.1 g |
| **Cholesterol** | 40 mg |
| **Sodium** | 500 mg |
| **Potassium** | 560 mg |
| **Total Carbohydrate** | 23 g |
| Dietary Fiber | 4 g |
| Sugars | 4 g |
| Added Sugars | 1 g |
| **Protein** | 19 g |
| **Phosphorus** | 230 mg |

# Meats and Fish

Even though chicken is one of the most commonly eaten proteins, there are other great meat options that are quick, easy, delicious, and can be very versatile in recipes, such as ground meats and fish fillets. Try these easy recipes with any of the starch or vegetable dishes in this book.

# Browned Ground Beef

## *(or any ground meat)*

SERVES 6 ■ SERVING SIZE 1/2 cup
PREP TIME 5 minutes ■ COOK TIME 20 minutes

Nonstick cooking spray

1 pound lean ground beef (90% lean)

**CHEF TIP**

You can use this method for any ground meat. It is especially important to ensure ground turkey and ground chicken are cooked through and no pink is left. Consuming raw or undercooked meats, poultry, seafood, shellfish, or eggs may increase your risk of foodborne illness.

## WAYS TO USE

- Mix with salsa and use as a filling for tacos, burritos, enchiladas, and quesadillas.
- Mix with sautéed tomatoes and bell peppers for sloppy joes.
- Season with a little salt and pepper and mix in with Scrambled Eggs (see page 54) and veggies.
- Add in to marinara sauce for a hearty pasta sauce.

1 Add the nonstick cooking spray to a nonstick skillet over high heat. Let the pan get hot, and then add the meat to the pan and break it into large pieces using a sturdy spatula or spoon. Let it brown for 5–6 minutes without touching it.

2 Using the spatula again, break the beef into smaller pieces as it cooks and browns. Try not to stir the beef too much; just stir occasionally until all of the beef is browned, another 8–10 minutes.

3 Cook until there is no pink meat left.

4 Drain any excess fat from the pan. Store in an airtight container for up to 1 week in the refrigerator or pack in freezer bags or containers for up to 3 months in the freezer.

**Choices/Exchanges**
2 Lean Protein

**Basic Nutritional Values**

| | | | |
|---|---|---|---|
| **Calories** | 120 | **Potassium** | 220 mg |
| Calories from Fat | 45 | **Total Carbohydrate** | 0 g |
| **Total Fat** | 6.0 g | Dietary Fiber | 0 g |
| Saturated Fat | 2.5 g | Sugars | 0 g |
| Trans Fat | 0.2 g | Added Sugars | 0 g |
| **Cholesterol** | 45 mg | **Protein** | 15 g |
| **Sodium** | 45 mg | **Phosphorus** | 130 mg |

# Simple Fish Fillets

**SERVES** 2 ■ **SERVING SIZE** 1 fillet
**PREP TIME** 5 minutes ■ **COOK TIME** 12–20 minutes
depending on the size of the fillet

Nonstick cooking spray

2 fresh or frozen fish fillets
(about 6 ounces each)
Options may include salmon,
cod, tilapia, haddock, or
flounder

2 teaspoons olive oil

1/4 teaspoon salt

1/4 teaspoon ground black
pepper

1 Preheat oven to 425°F for frozen
fillets or 375°F for fresh or thawed
fillets. Coat a baking sheet with
nonstick cooking spray and set
aside.

2 Pat the fillets dry with a paper towel
and then lightly brush both sides
with olive oil and season with salt
and pepper. If the fish has skin on it,
cook it skin-side-down. Note: You
can eat the skin or discard it after
cooking.

3 Place in the oven to bake.

4 Bake frozen fish for around
12–13 minutes for thin fillets and
15–17 minutes for thicker fillets.

5 Bake thawed fish at 375°F for
10 minutes for thin fillets and
18–20 minutes for thick fillets.

## CHEF TIP

Chef Tip: Fish should
be cooked to an internal temperature of 145°F. Serve with
Roasted Vegetable Salad (see
page 80).

**Choices/Exchanges (based on cod)**
4 1/2 very lean protein

**Nutrition Information (based on cod)**

| | | | |
|---|---|---|---|
| **Calories** | 200 | **Potassium** | 500 mg |
| Calories from Fat | 65 | **Total Carbohydrate** | 0 g |
| **Total Fat** | 7 g | Dietary Fiber | 0 g |
| Saturated Fat | 1.0 g | Sugars | 0 g |
| Trans Fat | 0.0 g | Added Sugars | 0 g |
| **Cholesterol** | 100 mg | **Protein** | 32 g |
| **Sodium** | 450 mg | **Phosphorus** | 585 mg |

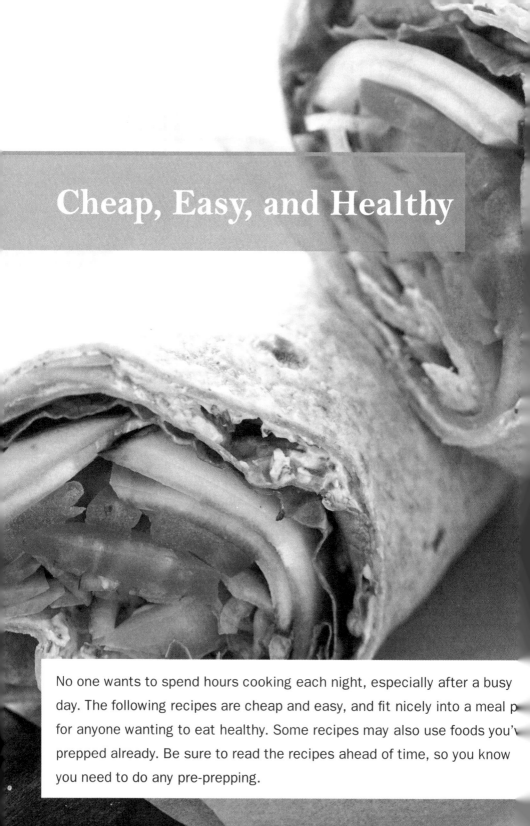

# Cheap, Easy, and Healthy

No one wants to spend hours cooking each night, especially after a busy day. The following recipes are cheap and easy, and fit nicely into a meal p for anyone wanting to eat healthy. Some recipes may also use foods you' prepped already. Be sure to read the recipes ahead of time, so you know you need to do any pre-prepping.

# Bean Burgers

SERVES 8 ■ SERVING SIZE 1 burger
PREP TIME 10 minutes ■ COOK TIME 15 minutes

3 cups cooked beans (see Cooked Dried Beans on page 73), or 2 (15-ounce) cans of any beans, drained and rinsed, divided, set aside

1/2 cup minced onion

1 cup cooked starch, such as brown rice, oatmeal, quinoa, or barley (see recipes on pages 58–71), set aside

1 large egg

1 teaspoon garlic powder

1/2 teaspoon salt

1/2 teaspoon ground black pepper

1 Add 1 1/2 cups of the beans to a large bowl with the onions. With a fork or potato masher, mash until mostly smooth (the mix will be slightly chunky because of the onions). Note: If you have a food processor, you can blend until smooth and then put in a bowl.

2 Add the remaining beans, the cooked starch, egg, garlic powder, salt, and pepper. Stir until well combined.

3 Form bean mixture into eight 1/2-inch-thick patties.

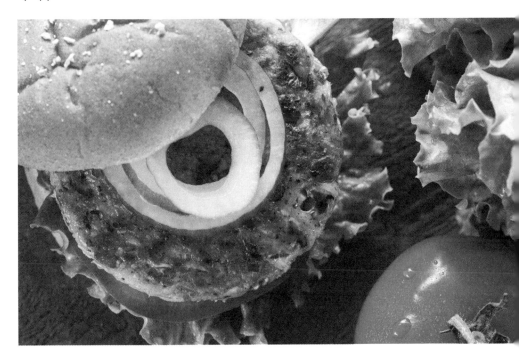

# Bean Burgers

*(continued)*

## WAYS TO USE

- Serve each bean burger in lettuce wrap topped with 1 Tablespoon salsa and an avocado slice.
- Use as a filling for a taco or burrito.
- Serve on a whole-grain bun with a slice of cheddar cheese, a large lettuce leaf, and a thick slice of tomato.

4 Add nonstick cooking spray to a nonstick skillet over medium heat. Add bean patties and cook about 2–3 minutes per side, until slightly brown. Work in batches if your pan is not big enough to hold all 8 burgers.

5 Store in an airtight container in the refrigerator for up to 1 week, or wrap individually in freezer bags or containers and freeze up to 6 months (freeze cooked burgers only; do not freeze the raw burgers).

**Choices/Exchanges**
1 1/2 Starch, 1 Lean Protein

**Basic Nutritional Values**

| | |
|---|---|
| **Calories** | 140 |
| Calories from Fat | 15 |
| **Total Fat** | 1.5 g |
| Saturated Fat | 0.4 g |
| Trans Fat | 0.0 g |
| **Cholesterol** | 25 mg |
| **Sodium** | 160 mg |
| **Potassium** | 330 mg |
| **Total Carbohydrate** | 24 g |
| Dietary Fiber | 6 g |
| Sugars | 1 g |
| Added Sugars | 0 g |
| **Protein** | 7 g |
| **Phosphorus** | 135 mg |

# Canned Protein Burger

**SERVES** 6 ■ **SERVING SIZE** 1 burger
**PREP TIME** 10 minutes ■ **COOK TIME** 15 minutes

2 (6-ounce) cans protein such as tuna, chicken, or salmon packed in water, drained

1/2 cup whole-grain breadcrumbs

1/4 cup light mayonnaise

1/4 cup minced onion

1/4 cup minced bell pepper

1 egg

1/2 teaspoon salt

1/2 teaspoon ground black pepper

1 Tablespoon olive oil

1  In a bowl, mix together the canned protein, breadcrumbs, light mayonnaise, onion, bell pepper, egg, salt, and pepper until combined.

2  Form into 6 patties.

3  Add olive oil to a nonstick skillet over medium heat. Fry burgers on each side for 3–4 minutes. Work in batches if your pan is not big enough to hold all 8 burgers.

4  Store in an airtight container in the refrigerator for up to 1 week, or wrap individually in freezer bags or containers and freeze up to 3 months (freeze cooked burgers only; do not freeze the raw burgers).

## WAYS TO USE

- Serve each burger in a lettuce wrap topped with 1 Tablespoon salsa and an avocado slice.
- Use as a filling for a taco or burrito.
- Serve on a whole-grain bun with a slice of cheddar cheese, a large lettuce leaf, and a thick slice of tomato.

## CHEF TIP

You can substitute the whole-grain breadcrumbs for a cooked starch such as brown rice, oatmeal, quinoa, or barley (see recipes on pages 58–71).

**Choices/Exchanges**
1/2 Starch, 1 Lean Protein, 1 Fat

**Basic Nutritional Values**

| | |
|---|---|
| **Calories** | 130 |
| Calories from Fat | 60 |
| **Total Fat** | 7.0 g |
| Saturated Fat | 0.9 g |
| Trans Fat | 0.0 g |
| **Cholesterol** | 50 mg |
| **Sodium** | 440 mg |
| **Potassium** | 140 mg |
| **Total Carbohydrate** | 8 g |
| Dietary Fiber | 1 g |
| Sugars | 1 g |
| Added Sugars | 0 g |
| **Protein** | 11 g |
| **Phosphorus** | 110 mg |

# Cheese and Veggie Wraps

SERVES 4 ■ SERVING SIZE 1 wrap
PREP TIME 10 minutes ■ COOK TIME 0 minutes

4 (7-inch) whole-wheat, low-carb tortillas

1/2 cup prepared hummus or Herby Bean Dip (see page 75)

1/4 cup shredded Pepper Jack cheese

1 medium red bell pepper, cut into 12 strips

4 large lettuce leaves

1/4 cup light ranch dressing or Creamiest Ranch Dressing (see page 86)

1 Lay one of the whole-grain flour tortillas on a cutting board. Spread with 2 Tablespoons hummus (or Herby Bean Dip), 1 Tablespoon Pepper Jack cheese, 3 strips of red bell pepper, 1 large lettuce leaf, and 1 Tablespoon ranch dressing (or Creamiest Ranch Dressing).

2 Roll the wrap from the bottom up, leaving the ends open.

3 Repeat for remaining 3 wraps.

4 These are best served immediately. If you only want one, save the rest of the ingredients for another day and make the wraps as needed.

**CHEF TIP**
Change up the flavors of this wrap with different cheeses, or try adding some Roasted Vegetables to it (see page 78).

**Choices/Exchanges**
1 Starch, 1 Nonstarchy Vegetable, 1 Lean Protein, 1 Fat

**Basic Nutritional Values**

| | |
|---|---|
| **Calories** | 170 |
| Calories from Fat | 90 |
| **Total Fat** | 10.0 g |
| Saturated Fat | 2.3 g |
| Trans Fat | 0.0 g |
| **Cholesterol** | 5 mg |
| **Sodium** | 520 mg |
| **Potassium** | 210 mg |
| **Total Carbohydrate** | 20 g |
| Dietary Fiber | 11 g |
| Sugars | 4 g |
| Added Sugars | 0 g |
| **Protein** | 10 g |
| **Phosphorus** | 165 mg |

# Mediterranean Sweet Potato Bowl

**SERVES** 1 ■ **SERVING SIZE** 1 bowl
**PREP TIME** 10 minutes ■ **COOK TIME** 5 minutes

1 cup cooked, cubed sweet potatoes (see Quick "Baked" Sweet Potatoes on page 83)

1/2 cup cooked 90% lean ground beef (see Browned Ground Beef on page 102)

Pinch of ground black pepper

1 Tablespoon chopped Kalamata olives

1 Tablespoon crumbled feta cheese

1/4 cup diced cucumber

1 Tablespoon red wine vinaigrette dressing (such as Wishbone) or Easy Vinaigrette (see page 85)

1 Reheat the sweet potatoes and the ground beef in separate bowls in the microwave for 30 seconds–1 minute.

2 Add the ground beef to the top of the sweet potatoes in a bowl. Top with the olives, feta cheese, and diced cucumber, and drizzle with the vinaigrette dressing. Serve immediately.

3 If packing to take for lunch, layer the cold sweet potatoes, ground beef, olives, and feta cheese in a microwave-safe to-go container. Store the cucumbers and vinaigrette separately in a small container. To reheat, heat the whole bowl in the microwave for 1 minute, then top with the cucumbers and vinaigrette to serve.

**Choices/Exchanges** ▬▬▬
2 1/2 Starch, 3 Lean Protein, 1 1/2 Fat

**Basic Nutritional Values** ▬▬▬

| | |
|---|---|
| **Calories** | 390 |
| Calories from Fat | 140 |
| **Total Fat** | 15.0 g |
| Saturated Fat | 4.6 g |
| Trans Fat | 0.3 g |
| **Cholesterol** | 65 mg |
| **Sodium** | 450 mg |
| **Potassium** | 1160 mg |
| **Total Carbohydrate** | 40 g |
| Dietary Fiber | 6 g |
| Sugars | 14 g |
| Added Sugars | 2 g |
| **Protein** | 24 g |
| **Phosphorus** | 295 mg |

# Hearty Grilled Cheese

SERVES 2 ■ SERVING SIZE 1/2 sandwich
PREP TIME 5 minutes ■ COOK TIME 10 minutes

1 Tablespoon reduced-fat cream cheese

2 Tablespoons shredded Monterey Jack cheese

1 Tablespoon fat-free, plain Greek yogurt

Pinch of ground black pepper

1/2 cup finely chopped Roasted Vegetables (see page 78), set aside

2 teaspoons light mayonnaise

2 slices whole-wheat sandwich bread

1 In a small bowl, mix together the cream cheese, Monterey Jack cheese, yogurt, and ground black pepper. Stir in the roasted vegetables. Set aside.

2 Spread 1 teaspoon light mayonnaise on one side of one piece of bread. Lay it mayonnaise-side-down in a nonstick skillet off the heat.

3 Spread the cheese and vegetable mixture on top of the piece of bread that is in the skillet. Top with the other piece of bread and spread the top of it with the remaining teaspoon of light mayonnaise.

4 Cook over low heat on the stovetop for 2 minutes. Then flip the sandwich to the other side and cook for 2 minutes. Continue to flip back and forth in 1-minute increments until both sides are dark golden brown and the filling is melted. Serve immediately.

## CHEF TIP

You can repeat this recipe for as many sandwiches as you want to make.

**Choices/Exchanges**
1 Starch, 1 Nonstarchy Vegetable, 1 Lean Protein, 1 Fat

**Basic Nutritional Values**

| | | | |
|---|---|---|---|
| **Calories** | 200 | **Potassium** | 250 mg |
| Calories from Fat | 70 | **Total Carbohydrate** | 24 g |
| **Total Fat** | 8.0 g | Dietary Fiber | 3 g |
| Saturated Fat | 2.7 g | Sugars | 6 g |
| Trans Fat | 0.0 g | Added Sugars | 3 g |
| **Cholesterol** | 15 mg | **Protein** | 9 g |
| **Sodium** | 350 mg | **Phosphorus** | 170 mg |

# Egg and Veggie Scramble

SERVES 2 ■ SERVING SIZE 3/4 cup
PREP TIME 5 minutes ■ COOK TIME 10 minutes

2 large eggs

2 large egg whites

2 Tablespoons fat-free, plain Greek yogurt

1/4 teaspoon salt

Pinch of ground black pepper

2 teaspoons olive oil

1 small onion, peeled and small diced

1 red bell pepper, small diced

1. In a medium bowl, whisk together the whole eggs, egg whites, yogurt, salt, and pepper. Set aside.

2. Add the olive oil to a nonstick skillet over medium heat.

3. Add the onion and bell pepper to the pan and sauté for 4–5 minutes, or until vegetables start to soften.

4. Pour the egg mixture into the pan and, with a wooden spoon or heatproof rubber spatula, scrape the bottom of the pan slowly and continuously until the eggs are set and not runny. Remove from heat and serve immediately.

**CHEF TIP**
This recipe is great on its own, but can also be served in a warm whole-grain tortilla with some hot sauce, or on toast topped with a little salsa.

**Choices/Exchanges**
2 Nonstarchy Vegetable, 1 Lean Protein, 2 Fat

**Basic Nutritional Values**

| | |
|---|---|
| **Calories** | 180 |
| Calories from Fat | 90 |
| **Total Fat** | 10.0 g |
| Saturated Fat | 2.2 g |
| Trans Fat | 0.0 g |
| **Cholesterol** | 185 mg |
| **Sodium** | 430 mg |
| **Potassium** | 370 mg |
| **Total Carbohydrate** | 10 g |
| Dietary Fiber | 2 g |
| Sugars | 6 g |
| Added Sugars | 0 g |
| **Protein** | 13 g |
| **Phosphorus** | 155 mg |

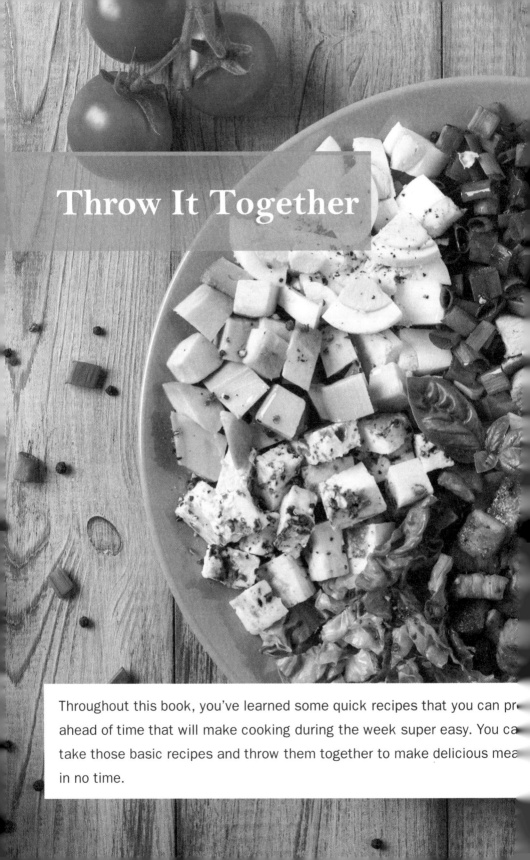

# Throw It Together

Throughout this book, you've learned some quick recipes that you can pr[e]
ahead of time that will make cooking during the week super easy. You ca[n]
take those basic recipes and throw them together to make delicious mea[ls]
in no time.

# Veggie, Bean, and Rice Taco Skillet

SERVES 8 ■ SERVING SIZE 1/2 cup
PREP TIME 5 minutes ■ COOK TIME 10 minutes

1 1/2 cups Roasted Vegetables (see page 78)

1 1/2 cups cooked beans (see Cooked Dried Beans on page 73), or 1 15-ounce can of beans, drained and rinsed

1 cup cooked Brown Rice (see page 59)

1/2 teaspoon ground black pepper

1 teaspoon ground cumin

1 Tablespoon chili powder

1 cup salsa

1/2 cup shredded Monterey Jack cheese

1 Combine all of the ingredients except the cheese in a nonstick skillet over medium heat. Cook for 7–8 minutes, stirring occasionally, until everything is heated through.

2 Sprinkle the cheese over the top of the mixture and let it melt (1–2 minutes) then serve.

3 Store cooled leftovers in an airtight container in the refrigerator for up to 1 week.

## WAYS TO USE

- Eat on its own with a side salad.
- Serve in whole-grain or corn tortillas as tacos.
- Serve in lettuce cups.
- Serve over whole-grain tortilla chips as nachos.

**Choices/Exchanges**
1 Starch, 1 Nonstarchy Vegetable, 1/2 Fat

**Basic Nutritional Values**

| | |
|---|---|
| **Calories** | 140 |
| Calories from Fat | 40 |
| **Total Fat** | 4.5 g |
| Saturated Fat | 1.7 g |
| Trans Fat | 0.0 g |
| **Cholesterol** | 5 mg |
| **Sodium** | 270 mg |
| **Potassium** | 390 mg |
| **Total Carbohydrate** | 20 g |
| Dietary Fiber | 5 g |
| Sugars | 3 g |
| Added Sugars | 0 g |
| **Protein** | 6 g |
| **Phosphorus** | 155 mg |

# Big Hearty Salad

SERVES 1 ■ SERVING SIZE 1 salad
PREP TIME 10 minutes ■ COOK TIME 0 minutes

1 cup baby salad greens

1/4 cup cooked barley (see Basic Barley on page 68)

1/4 cup cooked shredded chicken (see recipes on pages 95–100)

1 cup assorted chopped vegetables such as cucumber, bell pepper, carrots, and celery

1 Tablespoon toasted slivered almonds

1 hard-boiled egg, quartered (see Hard-Boiled Eggs on page 51)

2 Tablespoons Easy Vinaigrette (see page 85)

1 In a soup bowl, lay the 1 cup salad greens on the bottom of the bowl. Sprinkle the greens with the 1/4 cup cooked barley.

2 Sprinkle the 1/4 cup cooked, shredded chicken over the barley and top with the cut-up vegetables.

3 Sprinkle the slivered almonds over the vegetables, and then arrange the 4 egg slices around the edge of the salad.

4 Drizzle the 2 Tablespoons of vinaigrette over the whole salad.

## CHEF TIP

Make this to go! In a large mason jar, put the vegetables in the bottom of the jar and pour the 2 Tablespoons of dressing over them. Layer in this order on top of the vegetables: chicken, barley, eggs, cheese, almonds, and salad greens. When it's time to eat, simply shake the jar to distribute all of the ingredients, and eat right out of the jar.

Choices/Exchanges
1 Starch, 2 Nonstarchy Vegetable, 2 Lean Protein, 5 Fat

**Basic Nutritional Values**

| | |
|---|---|
| **Calories** | 460 |
| Calories from Fat | 270 |
| **Total Fat** | 30.0 g |
| Saturated Fat | 5.2 g |
| Trans Fat | 0.0 g |
| **Cholesterol** | 215 mg |
| **Sodium** | 200 mg |
| **Potassium** | 670 mg |
| **Total Carbohydrate** | 25 g |
| Dietary Fiber | 7 g |
| Sugars | 8 g |
| Added Sugars | 3 g |
| **Protein** | 22 g |
| **Phosphorus** | 295 mg |

# Purple Berry Salad

SERVES 2 ■ SERVING SIZE 3/4 cup
PREP TIME 10 minutes ■ COOK TIME 0 minutes

1/2 cup fresh raspberries

1/2 cup fresh blueberries

1/2 cup fresh blackberries

1/4 cup fat-free vanilla yogurt
(Greek-style or regular)

1 teaspoon lemon juice

1 Toss all ingredients gently together in a bowl. Serve immediately.

## CHEF TIP

Try making your own vanilla yogurt! Start with plain fat-free yogurt (Greek or regular) and sweeten to taste with honey, maple syrup, or granulated sugar substitute such as Stevia. Add a small splash of vanilla extract and stir to combine.

**Choices/Exchanges**
1 Fruit

**Basic Nutritional Values**

| | |
|---|---|
| **Calories** | 70 |
| Calories from Fat | 5 |
| **Total Fat** | 0.5 g |
| Saturated Fat | 0.1 g |
| Trans Fat | 0.0 g |
| **Cholesterol** | 0 mg |
| **Sodium** | 15 mg |
| **Potassium** | 170 mg |
| **Total Carbohydrate** | 15 g |
| Dietary Fiber | 5 g |
| Sugars | 8 g |
| Added Sugars | 1 g |
| **Protein** | 2 g |
| **Phosphorus** | 45 mg |

# "Leftovers" Hash

SERVES 2 ■ SERVING SIZE about 1 3/4 cup hash topped with 1 egg
PREP TIME 10 minutes ■ COOK TIME 10 minutes

Nonstick cooking spray

2 eggs

2 pinches (1/16 teaspoon) salt

1 Tablespoon water

1 cup cooked, cubed sweet potatoes (see Quick "Baked" Sweet Potatoes on page 83)

1 (3-ounce) chicken sausage (any flavor), medium diced (such as Al Fresco Sweet Italian Chicken Sausage)

2 cups Roasted Vegetables (see page 78)

1 clove garlic, minced or grated

1/2 teaspoon ground black pepper

1 Add nonstick cooking spray to a nonstick skillet over medium heat. Crack the two eggs into the skillet and sprinkle each with a pinch of salt. Pour the 1 Tablespoon water into the pan and cover for 4 minutes, or until the yolks of the eggs are set and the whites are firm. Slide the eggs on to a plate and set aside (cover with foil or another plate to keep warm).

2 In the same skillet, add more nonstick cooking spray and add the remaining ingredients. Sauté for 5-8 minutes, stirring occasionally until everything is heated through.

3 Divide the hash on two plates and top each with one egg.

## WAYS TO USE

Use any leftover ingredients you have for this dish such as:
- Easy Turkey Chili (see page 119) mixed with cooked whole-wheat pasta and Roasted Vegetables (see page 78); or
- Scrambled Eggs (see page 54), with Quick "Baked" Sweet Potatoes (see page 83) and Cooked Dried Beans (see page 73). Leave off the fried egg if using Scrambled Eggs and top with a little cheese instead.

Choices/Exchanges
1 Starch, 3 Nonstarchy Vegetable, 1 Medium Fat Protein, 2 Fat

| Basic Nutritional Values | |
|---|---|
| **Calories** | 310 |
| Calories from Fat | 140 |
| **Total Fat** | 15.0 g |
| Saturated Fat | 3.4 g |
| Trans Fat | 0.0 g |
| **Cholesterol** | 215 mg |
| **Sodium** | 590 mg |
| **Potassium** | 880 mg |
| **Total Carbohydrate** | 29 g |
| Dietary Fiber | 6 g |
| Sugars | 11 g |
| Added Sugars | 1 g |
| **Protein** | 18 g |
| **Phosphorus** | 300 mg |

# Simple Smoothie

SERVES 2 ■ SERVING SIZE 1 smoothie
PREP TIME 5 minutes ■ COOK TIME 0 minutes

1/2 cup frozen fruit (any)

1/2 medium banana

2 Tablespoons frozen chopped spinach

1 Tablespoon natural peanut or other nut butter

1 cup 1% low-fat milk

1/4 cup fat-free, plain Greek yogurt

1 Add all ingredients to a blender and purée until smooth.

2 Divide smoothie equally between 2 glasses. Serve immediately.

## CHEF TIP

If you are buying fresh fruit in season, wash, pat dry, and portion it into freezer bags so that you have peak-season fruit all year long.

**Choices/Exchanges**
1 Fruit, 1/2 Fat-Free Milk,
1 Lean Protein, 1/2 Fat

**Basic Nutritional Values**

| | |
|---|---|
| **Calories** | 170 |
| Calories from Fat | 50 |
| **Total Fat** | 6.0 g |
| Saturated Fat | 1.5 g |
| Trans Fat | 0.0 g |
| **Cholesterol** | 10 mg |
| **Sodium** | 70 mg |
| **Potassium** | 440 mg |
| **Total Carbohydrate** | 21 g |
| Dietary Fiber | 3 g |
| Sugars | 14 g |
| Added Sugars | 0 g |
| **Protein** | 10 g |
| **Phosphorus** | 200 mg |

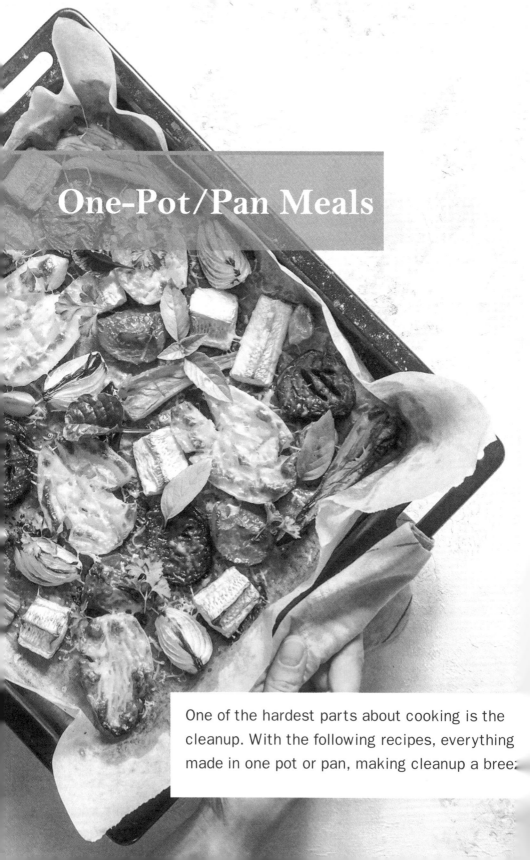

# One-Pot/Pan Meals

One of the hardest parts about cooking is the cleanup. With the following recipes, everything made in one pot or pan, making cleanup a breeze.

# Easy Turkey Chili

SERVES 4 ■ SERVING SIZE 1 1/4 cups
PREP TIME 10 minutes ■ COOK TIME 25 minutes

Nonstick cooking spray

1 pound lean ground turkey (93% lean, 7% fat)

1 bell pepper (any color), small diced

1 small yellow onion, peeled and small diced

1 14.5-ounce can no-salt-added diced tomatoes

1 Tablespoon chili powder

1 teaspoon cumin

1/2 teaspoon salt

1/2 teaspoon ground black pepper

*Optional ingredient:*

1/2 teaspoon cayenne pepper (to add more spice and flavor)

1 Heat a stock pot over high heat, then spray with nonstick cooking spray. Add the turkey and brown until just cooked through, about 7–8 minutes, stirring and breaking up the turkey as it cooks.

2 Add the remaining ingredients to the pot. Stir to combine, then bring to a boil over high heat. Reduce to a simmer and cook uncovered for 15 minutes, stirring occasionally.

3 Store cooled leftovers in an airtight container in the refrigerator for up to 1 week, or freeze 1-serving portions in freezer bags or containers for up to 3 months.

## WAYS TO USE

- Bulk this chili up by adding cooked beans (see Cooked Dried Beans on page 73) or grains such as cooked brown rice, quinoa, or barley (see recipes on pages 58–71), or whole-grain pasta.
- Serve on top of a baked sweet potato (see Quick "Baked" Sweet Potatoes on page 83).
- Use in "Leftovers" Hash (see page 116).
- Serve on top of whole-grain tortilla chips topped with a little shredded cheese, lettuce, and guacamole for nachos.

Choices/Exchanges
2 Nonstarchy Vegetable, 3 Lean Protein, 1 Fat

| Basic Nutritional Values | |
| --- | --- |
| **Calories** | 220 |
| Calories from Fat | 80 |
| **Total Fat** | 9.0 g |
| Saturated Fat | 2.6 g |
| Trans Fat | 0.1 g |
| **Cholesterol** | 85 mg |
| **Sodium** | 440 mg |
| **Potassium** | 610 mg |
| **Total Carbohydrate** | 10 g |
| Dietary Fiber | 3 g |
| Sugars | 5 g |
| Added Sugars | 0 g |
| **Protein** | 23 g |
| **Phosphorus** | 260 mg |

# Veggie and Barley Soup

SERVES 4 ■ SERVING SIZE 1 1/4 cups
PREP TIME 10 minutes ■ COOK TIME 20 minutes

1 12-ounce bag frozen California blend (cauliflower, carrots, and broccoli) vegetable medley

1 small onion, medium diced

1 clove garlic, minced or grated

1 quart (4 cups) low-sodium vegetable or chicken broth

1 cup cooked barley

1 Tablespoon dried parsley

1/8 teaspoon salt

1/2 teaspoon ground black pepper

1 Add the frozen vegetables, onion, garlic, and broth to a stock pot over high heat. Bring to a boil and reduce to a simmer for 10 minutes.

2 Add the remaining ingredients and simmer for 10 more minutes.

3 Store cooled leftovers in an airtight container in the refrigerator for up to 1 week or freeze 1-serving portions in freezer bags or conatiners for up to 3 months.

## CHEF TIP

You can add 1 cup cooked protein to this, like diced or shredded chicken (see recipes on pages 95–100), or ground beef, turkey, or chicken (see Browned Ground Beef on page 102).

**Choices/Exchanges**
1 Starch, 1 Nonstarchy Vegetable

**Basic Nutritional Values**

| | |
|---|---|
| **Calories** | 100 |
| Calories from Fat | 0 |
| **Total Fat** | 0.0 g |
| Saturated Fat | 0.1 g |
| Trans Fat | 0.0 g |
| **Cholesterol** | 0 mg |
| **Sodium** | 240 mg |
| **Potassium** | 360 mg |
| **Total Carbohydrate** | 22 g |
| Dietary Fiber | 6 g |
| Sugars | 5 g |
| Added Sugars | 0 g |
| **Protein** | 3 g |
| **Phosphorus** | 165 mg |

# Sheet Pan Fajitas

**SERVES** 4 ■ **SERVING SIZE** 4 chicken strips, 1/4 of the vegetables
**PREP TIME** 10 minutes ■ **COOK TIME** 25 minutes

Nonstick cooking spray

2 teaspoons chili powder

1/2 teaspoon ground cumin

2 teaspoons garlic powder

1/2 teaspoon salt

1 teaspoon ground black pepper

1 pound boneless skinless chicken breasts, cut into 1/2-inch-thick strips (16 strips total)

2 bell peppers (any color), sliced into strips

1 medium yellow onion, peeled and sliced

1 Tablespoon olive oil

2 Tablespoons lime juice

1 Preheat oven to 425°F. Line a sheet pan with foil and coat with nonstick cooking spray. Set aside.

2 In a small bowl, whisk together chili powder, cumin, garlic powder, salt, and black pepper.

3 Spread the chicken, bell peppers, and onions in a single layer on the sheet pan. Drizzle with the oil, lime juice, and spices and toss with your hands or with tongs to coat. Bake for 25 minutes, or until everything is thoroughly cooked and starting to brown.

4 Serve or store in an airtight container in the refrigerator for up to 1 week.

## CHEF TIP

You can make this with 1 pound of shrimp, too. Peel and devein the shrimp before cooking and reduce the cooking time to 15 minutes.

## WAYS TO USE

- Serve traditionally with corn tortillas, avocado, tomatoes, and lettuce.
- Serve cold over salad greens for a fajita salad.
- Mix with cooked Brown Rice (see page 59) and top with lettuce, tomato, and avocado for a fajita bowl.

**Choices/Exchanges**
2 Nonstarchy Vegetable, 3 Lean Protein

**Basic Nutritional Values**

| | | |
|---|---|---|
| **Calories** | 200 | |
| Calories from Fat | 60 | |
| **Total Fat** | 7.0 | g |
| Saturated Fat | 1.3 | g |
| Trans Fat | 0.0 | g |
| **Cholesterol** | 65 | mg |
| **Sodium** | 370 | mg |
| **Potassium** | 450 | mg |
| **Total Carbohydrate** | 10 | g |
| Dietary Fiber | 3 | g |
| Sugars | 4 | g |
| Added Sugars | 0 | g |
| **Protein** | 25 | g |
| **Phosphorus** | 215 | mg |

# Sheet Pan Lemon Garlic Salmon and Green Beans

**SERVES** 4 ■ **SERVING SIZE** 1 fillet and 1/4 of the vegetables
**PREP TIME** 10 minutes ■ **COOK TIME** 25 minutes

Nonstick cooking spray

1 12-ounce bag frozen French-cut green beans

4 4-ounce frozen skinless salmon fillets

1 teaspoon garlic powder

1/2 teaspoon salt

1/2 teaspoon ground black pepper

1/4 cup lemon juice

1 Tablespoon olive oil

1 Preheat oven to 400°F. Line a sheet pan with foil and coat with nonstick cooking spray.

2 Layer the frozen green beans in a single layer on the sheet pan and top with the 4 salmon fillets, set 2 inches apart.

3 Sprinkle the salmon and green beans with the garlic powder, salt, pepper, lemon juice, and olive oil.

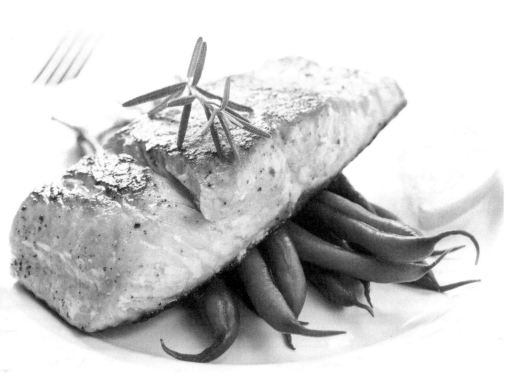

4  Bake in the oven for 25 minutes or until the internal temperature of the salmon is 145°F.*

5  Serve immediately or store in an airtight container in the refrigerator for up to 1 week.

## *COOKING SAFETY TIP

To take the internal temperature of fish, use an instant-read thermometer inserted into the thickest part of the fillet. You want to ensure that fish is cooked to 145°F (safe temperature of doneness for fish) before serving. Consuming raw or undercooked meats, poultry, seafood, shellfish, or eggs may increase your risk of foodborne illness.

**Choices/Exchanges**
1 Nonstarchy Vegetable, 3 Lean Protein, 1 1/2 Fat

**Basic Nutritional Values**

| | |
|---|---|
| **Calories** | 240 |
| Calories from Fat | 110 |
| **Total Fat** | 12.0 g |
| Saturated Fat | 2.4 g |
| Trans Fat | 0.0 g |
| **Cholesterol** | 60 mg |
| **Sodium** | 370 mg |
| **Potassium** | 520 mg |
| **Total Carbohydrate** | 8 g |
| Dietary Fiber | 2 g |
| Sugars | 1 g |
| Added Sugars | 0 g |
| **Protein** | 23 g |
| **Phosphorus** | 325 mg |

## CHEF TIP

Serve this with cooked Brown Rice (see page 59). You can use other types of fish, but if the fillets are thinner, reduce the cooking time to 18 minutes.

# One-Pot Cheesy Butternut Squash Soup

SERVES 8 ■ SERVING SIZE 3/4 cups
PREP TIME 10 minutes ■ COOK TIME 20 minutes

1 Tablespoon olive oil

1 pound frozen butternut squash cubes (*Note:* if you can't find these cubes frozen, try looking in the cut-up vegetables section in produce)

1 small onion, medium diced

1/2 teaspoon salt

1/2 teaspoon ground black pepper

8 ounces uncooked whole-wheat rotini pasta (about 3 cups uncooked pasta)

4 cups (1 quart) low-sodium chicken or vegetable broth

1/4 cup chopped fresh parsley

1/4 cup grated Parmesan cheese

1 Heat olive oil in a stock pot over medium-high heat. Add the butternut squash, onion, salt, and pepper and cook, stirring occasionally, until lightly browned, about 3 minutes.

2 Add uncooked pasta and broth and bring to a boil for 10 minutes.

3 Stir in parsley and cook another 5 minutes.

4 Stir in Parmesan cheese and serve.

5 Store cooled leftovers in an airtight container in the refrigerator for up to 1 week.

## CHEF TIP

If you have leftover shredded chicken (recipes on pages 95–100) or cooked beans (see Cooked Dried Beans on page 73), you can stir either into this dish for extra protein.

**Choices/Exchanges**
2 Starch, 1/2 Fat

**Basic Nutritional Values**

| | |
|---|---|
| **Calories** | 170 |
| Calories from Fat | 25 |
| **Total Fat** | 3.0 g |
| Saturated Fat | 0.7 g |
| Trans Fat | 0.0 g |
| **Cholesterol** | 0 mg |
| **Sodium** | 250 mg |
| **Potassium** | 460 mg |
| **Total Carbohydrate** | 29 g |
| Dietary Fiber | 4 g |
| Sugars | 3 g |
| Added Sugars | 0 g |
| **Protein** | 9 g |
| **Phosphorus** | 175 mg |

# Kale and Sausage Skillet with Brown Rice

SERVES 5 ▪ SERVING SIZE 1 cup
PREP TIME 10 minutes ▪ COOK TIME 15 minutes

1 Tablespoon olive oil

3 (3-ounce) fully cooked chicken sausage links (such as Johnsonville), any flavor (recommend Cajun flavor), large diced

1 small onion, medium diced (about 1 cup diced onion)

4 cups chopped kale (stems removed)

1/2 cup low-sodium chicken or vegetable broth

1/4 teaspoon salt

1/2 teaspoon ground black pepper

1 cup cooked Brown Rice (see page 59), set aside

1 Heat olive oil in a nonstick skillet over medium heat. Add diced sausage and onion and sauté until onions begin to turn golden brown, about 3-5 minutes

2 Add the kale and chicken broth and sauté for a few more minutes, until kale softens.

3 Add salt, pepper, and cooked brown rice and sauté 3–4 more minutes to heat the rice through, then serve immediately

4 Store cooled leftovers in an airtight container in the refrigerator for up to 1 week.

**Choices/Exchanges** —
1/2 Starch, 1 Nonstarchy Vegetable, 1 Lean Protein, 1 Fat

**Basic Nutritional Values** —

| | |
|---|---|
| **Calories** | 180 |
| Calories from Fat | 80 |
| **Total Fat** | 9.0 g |
| Saturated Fat | 2.1 g |
| Trans Fat | 0.0 g |
| **Cholesterol** | 35 mg |
| **Sodium** | 530 mg |
| **Potassium** | 520 mg |
| **Total Carbohydrate** | 15 g |
| Dietary Fiber | 2 g |
| Sugars | 2 g |
| Added Sugars | 1 g |
| **Protein** | 10 g |
| **Phosphorus** | 190 mg |

# CHAPTER 6

# Conversions and Substitutions

## MEASUREMENT CONVERSION CHARTS

| Gallons | Quarts | Pints | Cups | Fluid Ounces |
|---------|--------|-------|------|--------------|
| 1 | 4 | 8 | 16 | 128 |
| 1/2 | 2 | 4 | 8 | 64 |
| 1/4 | 1 | 2 | 4 | 32 |
| 1/8 | 1/2 | 1 | 2 | 16 |

| Cups | Tablespoons | Teaspoons |
|------|-------------|-----------|
| 1 | 16 | 48 |
| 1/2 | 8 | 24 |
| 1/4 | 4 | 12 |
| 1/16 | 1 | 3 |
| | 1/2 | 1 1/2 |

## SUBSTITUTES

For 1 whole egg in baking, substitute:

- 1 Tablespoon ground flaxseed + 3 Tablespoons water
- 1/2 medium banana, mashed
- 1/4 cup (4 Tablespoons) apple sauce
- 1/4 cup (4 Tablespoons) plain yogurt
- 1/4 cup (4 Tablespoons) buttermilk

For sour cream, substitute:

- Fat-free, plain Greek yogurt

For mayonnaise, substitute:

- 1/2 light mayonnaise, 1/2 fat-free, plain Greek yogurt

For breadcrumbs, substitute:

- Oats

For all-purpose flour, substitute:

- 1/2 of the all-purpose flour with whole-wheat flour

For white rice, substitute:

- Brown rice
- Barley
- Quinoa
- Oatmeal

For white pasta, substitute:

- Whole-wheat or whole-grain pasta
- Brown rice
- Barley
- Quinoa
- Oatmeal
- Spiralized vegetables
- Spaghetti squash

For canned beans, substitute:

- 1 1/2 cups  drained cooked dried beans

For buttermilk, substitute:

- 1 cup 1% low-fat milk and 1 Tablespoon lemon juice

# Index

Steel-Cut Oats, 61, 63
Stir-Fries
Chicken and Veggie Stir-Fry, 98–99
Veggie and Oatmeal Stir-Fry, 65
Stock pots, 6
Storage. *See* Food storage
Stuffed vegetables, Barley-Stuffed
Peppers, 70–71
Substitutions, 127–128
for increasing fiber, 34
for lowering calories and fat, 34
for lowering carbohydrates, 33
of vegetables for starches, 31–33
Sugars
added vs. natural, 20
healthier swaps for, 33
on nutrition labels, 20
Supplemental Nutrition Assistance
Program (SNAP), 16, 22
Sweet potatoes
Mediterranean Sweet Potato Bowl,
109
Quick "Baked" Sweet Potatoes, 83
Sweeteners, 21

Tea, 30
Temperature. *See* Internal temperature
Thawing foods, 10, 46–47
Thermometer, 11. *See also* Internal
temperature
Tomatoes, storing, 42
Tools, essential kitchen, 5–7
Turkey
Browned Ground Turkey, 102
Easy Turkey Chili, 119
internal temperature of, 11

U.S. Department of Agriculture (USDA)
Food and Nutrition Service of, 23
on food safety, 11, 48
MyPlate Kitchen of, 2
SNAP program of, 22
Utensils, 7

Vegetables, 76–83. *See also specific
vegetables*
buying fresh, frozen, or canned,
16–18
freezing, 44–45
healthier swaps for salt on, 35
nonstarchy, 26–27
peeling, 41–42
preparing ahead, 39, 40–42
as proportion of plate, 26–27, 29
raw, 39, 77
roasted, 77–80
spiralized, 31–32, 33
starchy, 29
storing, 42–43
as substitute for starches, 31–32
washing, 40–41
Veggie, Bean, and Rice Taco Skillet,
113
Veggie and Barley Soup, 120
Veggie and Oatmeal Stir-Fry, 65
Videos, YouTube, 2–3, 42
Vinaigrette, Easy, 85

Washing. *See* Cleaning
Water, drinking, 30
Websites, 2–3
White bread, healthier swaps for, 34
White rice, healthier swaps for, 34,
128
Whole grains, 21
Whole milk, healthier swaps for, 34
Whole Roasted Chicken, 90–91
Wraps. *See also* Sandwiches
Cheese and Veggie Wraps, 108
Chicken Lettuce Wraps, 97
healthier swaps for, 33

Yogurt, 115
YouTube, 2–3, 42

Zucchini, spiralized, 31–32, 33